The
Sisterhood
of **Diabetes**

Facing Challenges & Living Dreams

Judith Jones-Ambrosini

KALINDI PRESS
Chino Valley, Arizona

Cover Design: Adi Zuccarello

Interior Design and Layout: Becky Fulker, Kubera Book Design, Prescott, Arizona

Library of Congress Cataloging-in-Publication Data

Jones-Ambrosini, Judith, author.
  The sisterhood of diabetes : facing challenges and living dreams / Judith Jones-Ambrosini.
     pages cm
  Includes bibliographical references and index.
  ISBN 978-1-935826-34-7 (trade pbk. : alk. paper)
  1. Diabetes. 2. Diabetes--Miscellanea. 3. Diabetics--Counseling of. I. Title.
  RC660.J55 2014
  616.4'62--dc23
                           2013049116

Kalindi Press (an affiliate of Hohm Press)
P.O. Box 4410
Chino Valley, AZ 86323
800-381-2700
http://www.kalindipress.com

This book was printed in the U.S.A. on recycled, acid-free paper using soy ink.

Disclaimer:
It is not the intent of the author or any of the interviewed athletes to diagnose or prescribe, nor is the purpose of this book to replace the services of a competent physician. The material is intended for educational and motivational purposes only. It is advisable to seek the services of a licensed, professional healthcare provider for any condition that may require medical or psychological services.

Praise for *The Sisterhood of Diabetes*

"Amazing" best describes the women in this book. Ambrosini illustrates, again and again, that the only limitations from living with diabetes are those we impose upon ourselves. Her brief explanation of diabetes care in the 1960s, when she was diagnosed, will be fascinating to those familiar with current care. *Sisterhood* is a great source of inspiration and motivation to women living with diabetes.

–**Jeff Hitchcock,** founder: Children with Diabetes (CWD)

Judith's book brilliantly captures these sisters' courage, indomitable spirit and unwavering willingness to do what it takes to manage diabetes, exercise and sport. If you are a woman with diabetes, love a woman with diabetes, or are involved in the health care of women with diabetes *The Sisterhood of Diabetes* is truly a remarkable and necessary read.

–**Matthew H. Corcoran, MD,** CDE; CEO and founder:
Diabetes Training Camp

For all parents of diabetic children, Judith Jones-Ambrosini's book answers the questions they need answered. My son Jordan decided to stop playing athletics when he was diagnosed, but to all future athletes with diabetes, the world can be your oyster. That hope emanates from Judith's tome.

–**Ron Darling,** former Major League Baseball player; Emmy Award
winning broadcaster; Jordan Darling's (Type 1 diabetes) father

These inspiring profiles in courage not only give hope to those with diabetes but to anyone facing physical or emotional challenges preventing them from a full and rewarding life. I know many of the women in this sisterhood, including the author, and yet I came away with a profound and renewed sense of awe and respect. Reading their stories makes me yearn for a brotherhood of diabetes.

–**Charles Renfroe**, Director of Advocacy & Alliances,
Johnson & Johnson Diabetes Solutions

It's about time someone gave credit where credit is due. The remarkable women described in this book are breaking new ground and serving as inspiration for generations to come. Judith Jones-Ambrosini does an outstanding job of telling their stories and sharing their secrets to success.

–**Gary Scheiner**, MS, CDE; owner and clinical director:
Integrated Diabetes Services, LLC; author, *Think Like A Pancreas*;
2014 AADE Diabetes Educator of the Year

Praise for *The Sisterhood of Diabetes*

This "sisterhood" is comprised of strong, supportive women who actively chose to embrace their diabetes in order to help them live out their dreams. *The Sisterhood of Diabetes* can motivate and encourage anyone living with diabetes to overcome the challenges they face in their self-care. *What's not to love about that?!*

> – **Max "Mr. Divabetic" Szadek**, founder of Divabetic, a multimedia educational organization for women with diabetes

This book is about women with diabetes doing extraordinary things, not *because* of their diabetes, but *in spite of it*. The life stories of these impressive athletes prove that the best lives are lived out loud, without self-imposed boundaries.

> –**Victor Van Beuren**, MS, American Diabetes Association, Senior Manager: Acquisitions, ADA Books

The experience, wisdom, and heart Judith has put into this book is guaranteed to benefit and inspire all who read it. It's amazing to see so many stories of successful women living with diabetes all in one place. Personally, Judith is someone who I have always admired, and is one of the most genuine warm hearted persons I have ever met.

> – **Phil Southerland**, president, founder, and Chairman of the Board: Team Type 1; Director of Health Care Policy, Planning and Patient Advocacy–WHO Collaborating Center, International Diabetes Center and Mayo Clinic

Judith's collection of notable women with diabetes who exercise in creative ways inspires, enthralls, entertains and raises every reader's motivation to move. As a member of the Sisterhood, Judith tells their stories from an experienced insider's point of view.

> –**Ruth Roberts**, MA, and **John Walsh**, PA, CDE, authors of *Pumping Insulin* and *Using Insulin*

For
Janie Jones and Danny Ambrosini

Guardian Angel
Guiding Light

They play hard, move fast, and seek out challenges. They carry their diabetes with them every step of the way. Their energy whirls and emerges with spins to inspire all of us.

—Judith Jones-Ambrosini

Contents

Preface

Bruce Perkins, MD, MPH

Division of Endocrinology and Metabolism, Department of Medicine, University of Toronto, Canada

The year that I was diagnosed with diabetes was the year that a certain film, called *Steel Magnolias,* was released. This film was disproportionately troubling to me, much more than a typical Hollywood comedy-drama should be. Though on its surface it was about the strength of women and their undying support of one another in a southern American town, at its heart it was a movie about the devastating nature of diabetes—in particular, how it could insidiously ruin a woman in her prime. This was not the diabetes that I had just learned about, the diabetes that I thought I could handle, that I could reconcile within an adventurous, happy, ambitious and accomplished life. Rather, it was the kind of diabetes marred by limits—by convulsive low blood sugar attacks, by progressive kidney failure in pregnancy. It showed the contradictions of a beautiful young woman who was, because of her diabetes, forced to live life hesitantly and to meet its exciting milestones with fear. Without question, this movie influenced a generation of women with diabetes, who grew up with an uncomfortable fear over bearing children, over having families of their own, over pursuing the elements of a full and rewarding life. The death of the key character, Shelby, represented for me the end of that apparently naïve notion that a life with diabetes could be completely limitless and free of a sense of fear—particularly if you were a woman with diabetes.

How I was wrong! The fundamental task once diagnosed with diabetes is to eventually raise your chin, grit your teeth, be organized and headstrong and move forward. Don't just pursue your dreams, but pursue them like the Sisters in this book—reconciled with determination balanced with a healthy respect for diabetes. Having met many of these Sisters, I came to learn that in this day and age—in an era where we have effective insulin preparations, pump therapy, better ways to test for the development of early complications, measure our blood sugars, and ways to use new technologies creatively—a person with diabetes can lead a life in parallel to a life without diabetes. With adequate knowledge and motivation, one can lead a life just as challenging, as adventurous, as ambitious, and as inspirational. The key to accomplishing this is held collectively within the stories that you will read in this book.

What do the Sisters in this book have in common? They have all used exercise or sports in some way as a countermeasure to the stress imposed by diabetes. They either inspire us to the possibilities of what we can accomplish physically—or they teach us a specific lesson about how we can manage exercise safely—despite our diabetes. I had to wonder, though, why the Sisters emphasized so much their accomplishments in exercise and sport. After all, there are so many different ways that we can uniquely express ourselves and overcome the limits of diabetes. Then it struck me—to the body with diabetes, exercise poses a specific set of challenges that, if understood, teach us to manage any challenge in life. If one can understand the particular blood sugar patterns and necessary insulin adjustments to run a marathon, swim the Atlantic, race horses, excel on the ice, then there is no challenge in life that cannot be overcome. These accomplishments prepare us to successfully survive college exams, travel the world, be politically active, fly a plane, motivate a crowd through song, or paint a masterpiece! In short, the lessons learned through exercise and sport help us with life, to pursue our passions, and to develop our world view—all through helping us with the task of better managing our own diabetes.

Unfortunately, exercise and diabetes represent a challenging combination. In the medical field, we know that exercise and sports are extremely important for our psychological well-being and the development of our social skills for individual success and for teamwork. Exercise improves our physical fitness, helps us to maintain a healthy weight, control our blood pressure and cholesterol, and lower our risk for heart attacks and strokes. On the other hand, despite all of these benefits that we can derive from exercise, research studies that have specifically looked at improving blood sugar control—especially in those with Type 1 (or "juvenile onset") diabetes—do not consistently show benefit from exercise. These studies have shown us that the risk of low blood sugar reactions are often increased by exercise, that we can develop troublesome blood sugar elevations following high-impact exercise. In some of these studies, the overall blood sugar control of many participants was even worsened by taking part in an exercise program. If exercise has so many positive attributes, why is it that it was not naturally helpful in those diabetes clinical research studies? The answer is because successful exercise requires in-depth knowledge about exercise, about diabetes itself, and about taking the time to learn about one's own unique blood-sugar patterns during different types of exercise.

The body has a set of well-tuned mechanisms to control the fuels that we need for energy—including blood sugar—during exercise. This fine balance is thrown off in those with diabetes who are taking insulin therapy. To prevent the low and high blood sugar swings associated with exercise, those with diabetes must learn the details of what their own bodies would do if they did not have diabetes, in order to time ingesting sugar and carbohydrates, and making adjustments in insulin. For example, during typical "aerobic" exercise—such as running, swimming, dancing, cycling—muscles for the first minutes can use stored energy within the muscle cells as fuel. Not too long afterward, though, those cells need to start pulling energy—including sugar—from the blood, risking a dangerous drop in the level of blood sugar. The pancreas would normally notice this immediately, decrease (but not abolish) the amount of insulin put into the blood, and help to increase the levels of other "counter-insulin" hormones such as glucagon and stress hormones. Together, the decrease in insulin and increase in these latter hormones signal the liver—the body's main warehouse for storing sugar—to meticulously replace the sugar that the muscles have taken from the blood. The person on insulin therapy, though, often has relatively too much insulin floating in the blood to allow for safe exercise, so the liver is shut off from replacing the muscles' demands. The consequence—a low blood sugar reaction. To counteract this, people with diabetes learn about the quantity and timing of taking extra sugar by mouth, rather than relying fully on the liver. However, a decrease in insulin dose—for example the "basal," or background, insulin delivered through an insulin pump—can be adjusted in the hours before aerobic exercise to allow the liver to get involved by releasing stored sugar. Too much of a reduction in basal insulin puts a patient at risk of developing high blood sugar levels that can dehydrate, or even worse lead to the production of dangerous ketone bodies that can be life-threatening. Above all of this, "anaerobic" exercise, the very high intensity exercise that leads to absolute exhaustion and the "lactic acid burn" that one feels in the muscles, can also lead to dramatic rises in blood sugars on account of the stress hormones that tell the liver to release too much sugar. The bottom line is that exercise in diabetes is complex—it requires a patient to gradually become familiar with all of the necessary elements of an effective knowledge-base in diabetes. Those research trials failed in that they tried to apply the same approach to all of the patients, rather than to teach them about the necessary motivation and unique self-management skills. It is in this regard that this book helps to fill an enormous gap in the literature—it will help people with diabetes learn vital lessons from the Sisters who have succeeded.

The man who wrote *Steel Magnolias*, Robert Harling, picked up his pen and began writing as a means to help cope with the death of his own sister, a sister with diabetes. In dealing with these emotions, he felt that it was fundamentally important to show both the tragedy of his sister's death, but also to show the way his characters used humor and lightheartedness to cope with life. The Sisters in this book live day-to-day with an element of fear—they imagine Shelby and the turns that life could take—but they put those fears in a healthy perspective, and they reveal to us in their stories the magical combination of intensely focused work and a pride for loving life to its fullest. Decades after first seeing the movie, my reverence and awe for the strong woman with diabetes is only strengthened. My notion that a life with diabetes can be completely limitless and free of a sense of fear has been revived. The Sisters that you are about to meet may have a physical vulnerability that makes them delicate—as a magnolia—but their perseverance in reconciling a life with diabetes is as tough as steel. ✄

Introduction

Thinking back, there have been several memorable moments over the fifty-year course of time I have been living with Type 1 diabetes. I'll tell you about a few of them and how they led to writing this book.

"Goobledeygooinkadadigga," a voice hovered over me rattling incomprehensible sounds. "Oh shut up!" I said to myself, eyes opening gingerly to see who was blabbering on like that. He and his voice soon became clear. He was a handsome man dressed in whites—hospital whites. Who was this guy? Where was I? I nodded a faint smile as I tried desperately to figure out what the hell I was doing in a hospital. The moment came when I realized I had pneumonia. Damn! I hoped it wasn't double pneumonia. I had been surfing in the chilly autumn waters of the mighty Atlantic and caught an awful cold that I couldn't seem to shake. It was making me pee all the time and get so thirsty that I'd raise my hand in class constantly to go to the water fountain.

Suddenly, with a caring glance, the guy in whites asked if anyone *else* in my family had diabetes. Stunned, I yawned and pretended to fall back asleep. He walked away from my bed. DIABETES! DIABETES! What the hell was he talking about?

What exactly is diabetes anyway?

Over the next couple of weeks I learned that I had been rushed to the hospital in ketoacidosis (DKA), diabetic coma. In those days of the early 1960s, this meant learning how to administer insulin shots by piercing an orange. I remember feeling sorry for that orange. The day before my release from the hospital, the endocrinologist (the guy in whites) suggested that I make a list of questions in order to help with the transition from hospital to home. I had only one pressing question which I blurted out: Would I still be able to eat hot fudge sundaes? The kind doctor smiled and shook his head *no*, meaning it was out of the question. I could feel my chin quiver and my heart sink simultaneously. When he left my room, which was now filled with flowers, stuffed animals, cards and colorful balloons, I began to cry. I cried buckets of tears. No more sweet hot fudge sundaes made with my two favorite ice cream flavors, coffee and chocolate. No more nuts sprinkled on top under the puffy cloud of whipped cream. Why bother to live? What kind of a life could this be with diabetes and without hot fudge sundaes?

That was over fifty years ago, in 1962, and I was a breakaway young teenager who didn't like the "diabetic diet" that was prescribed back then—the stone age, the ice age, the dark age of diabetes care. It was the time we weighed food, sterilized glass syringes and sharpened 25-guage steel needles. It was when we poured murky urine samples into test tubes. It was a time when diabetes was painful to manage.

Today if I wanted something like a hot fudge sundae, I'd be able to figure out how to adjust my carb/insulin ratios on my insulin pump and adjust exercise to go for it. But at the end of the day I'd rather eat a peach than finagle for that five minutes of empty calories and sugar. My dissatisfaction with the diabetes "exchange diet" of that time, combined with a youthful folly of getting whatever I wanted, steered me in the direction of a career in the food business.

Fresh food and meal time were a major part of growing up with a mother who was a great Polish cook. She and my eight aunts, the Szumilowski sisters, used to send us kids to the butcher shop to buy "casings" for them to make their own kielbasa. They also made duck soup, kluski (noodles), babka, goluomka and pirogi. They hunted wild mushrooms and picked fresh corn and apples from fields and orchards in upstate New York. No wonder the graham crackers and skimmed milk snack recommended in the diabetic "Exchange" diet were not for me. I eventually became a chef and ran my own "Natural Celebrations" catering business in New York City for over twenty years, where I served healthy foods in fresh, vibrant and creative ways to the Park Avenue crowd.

It wasn't that I went from Mama's Polish kitchen into an exclusive New York catering business immediately. There were many side journeys that took me through college as an English major, to working in film in Italy for five years, where I also learned the beauty and passion of food, to living on an organic farm commune in Massawippi in the Eastern Townships of Canada for two years. There we ground wheat berries to make flour for bread, gathered water in rain barrels, and cooked over a wood stove since there was no electricity or running water on the farm.

Through those years of adventure and challenges, I never knew anyone else who had diabetes, but I learned to always carry my diabetes with me in a safe place my back pocket. I learned how being active made me feel good and kept my blood sugars balanced. In Italy, I walked hundreds of steps every day, up and down the mountain, and swam in the clear waters of the Tyrannean Sea in the little village of Positano, south of Naples on the Amalfi Coast. As part of everyday survival in the cold Canadian winters, I chopped wood and snow shoed for transportation. Summers anywhere meant biking, walking, planting and harvesting a lush sustenance garden. In Canada, we dug a root cellar to store vegetables for the scarce winter months. During those years of living and traveling, sometimes halfway around the world, with diabetes and my little son Jude as my constant companions, there were some gripping moments.

I have been mistaken for a witch, drug addict, drunk and mystic because of my diabetes. Along the way I have come to understand that I could reach out and make dreams happen despite having a chronic condition like diabetes. That awareness and confidence garnered a friendship.

One ordinary morning when I woke up, tested my urine with Testape litmus paper and injected my daily shot of NPH insulin, I realized that this diabetes was not going to leave me alone. It wasn't going away. I would have to repeat a similar routine the following morning and many mornings after that. It was another of those ah-ha moments. I decided to become friends with my diabetes. Seems like a silly way to put it, calling diabetes a friend. What it really means is to have that positive attitude about life which encourages one to dream and set high goals despite diabetes. With limited diabetes education available so many years ago, I didn't have a wide scope of references at my fingertips. The friendship deal seemed to make sense though. Diabetes gives us a roster of guidelines and regulations. Food, medication and exercise are the bare bones of diabetes care—although exercise was never highlighted as vital. But, I always felt better when I moved, and my blood sugars reflected it. Some form of sport or activity became part of my everyday life. I felt that by respecting the diabetes tenants and encircling those with a positive attitude, chances were that life would be healthy and fulfilling.

By the mid-1980s I made two new discoveries: one was Sheldon Bleicher, MD (who I called "the Wizard"), the other was the American Diabetes Association. They both provided great awakenings for this diabetes hermit. Dr. Bleicher taught me new ways to manage my diabetes and sparked an interest in fine tuning my diabetes care. He was a taskmaster and I learned so much from him. He will always be "the Wizard" to me.

When I heard about an organization called The American Diabetes Association and took a Volunteer Educators' certificate course, I discovered that other people, real people, had diabetes too. I wasn't alone anymore. I dove in head first by organizing a health walk called "Fitness-A-Foot" in New York's Central Park. It was my first time out with a team of volunteers who were all Type 1s, at a time when charity walks had not yet come into fashion but exercise was becoming mainstream. Our team worked well together and planned a fabulous event for April 7, 1989.

That morning, I looked out my apartment window in Greenwich Village and rubbed my eyes, thinking my vision was cloudy and maybe I was having a reoccurrence of the peripheral diabetic retinopathy I had a brush with in the mid-1970s. Instead, it had snowed all night and the city was blanketed in the most beautiful white carpet of early spring snow.

In Central Park, thanks to the number-one best partner any Type 1 can have—my "Type 3" husband and support system Danny Ambrosini—we were able to secure generators to power our needs. Volunteers and walkers showed up with thermoses of hot tea and coffee, and thanks to Danny for engineering the generator, music bellowed from the loudspeakers. A Type 1 aerobics instructor led a high energy warm-up dance, and soon we forged ahead with the 5K walk/run to raise awareness of the importance of exercise for diabetes.

Participants cheerfully set out on the snowy trail when suddenly the snow subsided and brilliant sunshine blazed through, clearing the sky, to bless the two hundred Type 1s, Type 2s and their families and friends who came out to support the cause.

Our core group of volunteers for this signature event remained friends for many years. I continued to volunteer with the ADA for another year when I was invited to join the NY ADA affiliate board, and thus launched a new life into the diabetes community for which I will be ever grateful. After years of helping with walks, fundraising events, family symposia, library programs and comedy crusades I began to widen my scope. I had been writing a food column called "The Shore Palate" for a New Jersey newspaper and found that I was referencing diabetes in many of my columns as part of my mission to get people to pay attention to eating a healthy diet and being active with exercise and sports. It was during this period that I began writing for *Diabetes Interview* (now *Diabetes Health*) magazine. One day Scott King, then publisher of the paper, called and invited me to California to write a story about an upcoming diabetes conference in Mission Springs. The event was organized by a group known as IDAA (International Diabetic Athletes Association), founded by Type 1 athlete and marathon runner, Paula Harper.

Once there, I marveled at the group of approximately 150 athletes all of whom had diabetes. I was home. I became consumed by the activities, workshops and camaraderie of the group.

The year was 1996, and many of the athletes at the conference managed their diabetes with insulin pumps. Dr. Bleicher had been encouraging me to try a pump, but I couldn't quite make the commitment to jump across the seemingly deep chasm from good-old-reliable insulin shots, to the gold standard of insulin pump therapy. Learning about pumps and other technology at the IDAA conference bolstered my confidence to take the leap. Until then I felt that nothing could help control my diabetes better than the six or more daily insulin shots I was taking, the eight blood glucose checks I did everyday on my meter as a runner, and the vegetarian diet I had been enjoying since 1969. Soon after the conference I began pumping insulin and haven't looked back since. Insulin pump therapy is not a cure, and not the perfect answer for everyone but it surely has helped me in my diabetes management.

It's 2014 now, and the science, technology, psychology and socialization of diabetes have developed and advanced greatly since 1962 and my hot fudge sundae memories. There are now many high-quality diabetes websites, blogs, and athletic and educational organizations. I continue to write about living a healthy lifestyle and about daily activity with diabetes for several magazines and *www.diabetesnet.com*, where I offer two monthly columns: "Judith's Cyber Kitchen" and "MoTo Move" for Ruth Roberts and John Walsh (two of the friends I met at the first IDAA conferences in California).

For five years, during a ten-year term on the DESA (Diabetes Exercise and Sports Association) board of directors, I served as editor of a quarterly newsletter on diabetes, sports and exercise, *The DESA Challenge*. I was honored with a "Lilly for Life" award for journalism. I teach tai chi classes at Divabetics meetings in New York City, at Diabetes Sisters' conferences, TCOYD (Taking Control of Your Diabetes) conferences, and other diabetes events. I stay active with distance walking, cycling and lots of dance. My husband and I have been volunteering with Sports Central, at "Children With Diabetes" conferences for ten years. Observing how smart the kids are about recognizing low blood sugars and knowing how many carb grams they need to treat them, and seeing how they run around as happy and healthy as their non-diabetic brothers, sisters and friends is deeply enlightening.

We know that living everyday with diabetes is not always a cakewalk. However, now is a time when research and education are working hand in hand to improve the quality of our daily lives. Diabetes is something that makes those of us who live with it special people. We are disciplined, determined and responsible, and often have an intuitive understanding about life that others don't need to have. As you read through the pages of this book you'll get to know the outstanding women who all say, "Yes, I have diabetes; just watch what I can do!"

I'd like to quote something from Elise Zevitz—one of the young athletes whose story is found in Chapter 12, *The Upcoming Inspiration Generation.* She says: "Having diabetes is like driving a car with a manual transmission. You have more control, more involvement and more responsibility—just like the very best sports cars."

The inspiration to write this book came on a plane trip home from a "Diabetes and Exercise" conference held in Colorado Springs, Colorado in 2007. On the night when the Lifescan Athletic Achievement Awards were presented at the Olympic Training Center there, I looked around at the audience, scanning this group of amazing athletes who live their lives with strength, responsibility, humor, discipline and an almost uncontrollable urge to show the world that they can achieve and live their dreams despite diabetes. I focused on the young girls and women of all ages, who were there participating in sports and exercise, and holding prospects of endless possibilities, as Camille Izlar notes in

Chapter 3, "We can do anything we set our goals on, it just takes a little more planning."

This book needed to be written to sing out the praises of these dazzling muses who move amongst us, and to inspire you, the reader, whether you have diabetes or not. I think you'll love the way *The Sisterhood of Diabetes* makes you feel. It's bound to get you moving!

— Judith Jones-Ambrosini
   Type 1 Optimist

p.s.

Unable to resist the urge to feed people, I will leave you with a healthy "take-on-a-hike" snack to carry in your backpack as you hike, bike, climb and reach for the top of your world. I first made these cookies for a diabetes and sports conference in New York City in 2002. They are packed with a big nutritional bang.

Make a big batch and freeze for future outings. Pack them in zip lock bags to keep the crunch going.

When you do your own baking as I do, you know exactly what goes into the diabetes mix. Choose healthy and nutritious ingredients to reward yourself with after a successful sport or activity that keeps you inspired.

TAKE-ON-A-HIKE COOKIES (makes about 70 cookies)

Preheat oven to 350 degrees

½ cup canola oil

½ cup smooth peanut butter (freshly made)

1 cup brown sugar

2 large fresh eggs

½ cup low fat milk

2 cups whole wheat flour

1 tsp. baking soda

1 generous Tbs. ground cinnamon

2 cups oatmeal (not instant)

¼ cup toasted wheat germ

½ cup dried cherries, cranberries or apricots (diced)

1 cup toasted sliced almonds

Directions

1. With electric beater, mix oil, peanut butter, sugar, eggs and milk until smooth and well blended. This should take about 3 minutes.
2. Add remaining ingredients one at a time, or mix them together in a separate bowl and add all at once.
3. Line baking sheets with parchment or foil, and drop small walnut-sized cookies on the baking sheets. Leave in irregular shapes for a homey, rustic look.
4. Bake 15-20 minutes or until cookies begin to turn slightly golden brown.

NUTRITIONAL QUALITIES: serving = 2 cookies. CALORIES = 95, PROTEIN = 2.5 grams, FAT = 4.2 grams, CARBOHYDRATES = 12 grams

OPTIONAL ADDITION: stir in ½ cup dark chocolate chips. Changes in nutritional information: CALORIES 105, PROTEIN same, FAT = 5.2 grams, CARBOHYDRATES = 13 grams

CHAPTER 1

The Pioneer Women

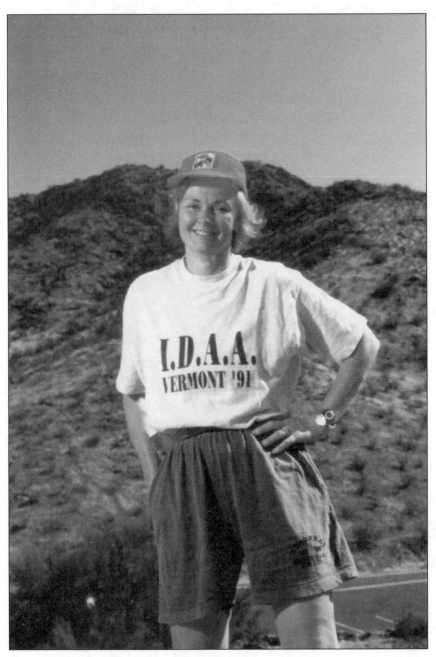

Paula Harper

PAULA HARPER

"I Run on Insulin"

It's a simple sentence formed with simple words. But these words were, in a sense, the "Big Bang," the spark that started the revolution in diabetes and exercise. When Paula Harper ran her first marathon in 1977, little did she know what was in store for her just a few years down the road. When first diagnosed with diabetes in 1972, routine medical advice was to avoid exercise. She was doing long-distance running, and got only negative or poor medical support for training and running pursuits. In the Phoenix marathon in the late 1970s, Paula wore a T-shirt that her husband Lew Harper had scribbled on with a magic marker. *I Run On Insulin* it read, on the back of the shirt. These words soon became the international call to arms for diabetes and exercise. The words echoed deeply on so many levels. Yes, Paula takes insulin, and she runs. Yes, insulin is the fuel that makes the machine work. And yes, a person can have diabetes and run marathons. The meaning of *I Run On Insulin* remains vital and potent to this day.

In Phoenix, Paula learned that she was not the only road warrior putting into practice something she instinctively believed in—the powerful tool of sports in helping to keep blood sugars managed. At that race, others came up to her with a sigh of relief to discover that they were no longer alone, reporting that they were also doing "trial and error" therapy. Through those common bonds of diabetes and exercise, they became comrades and friends. They exchanged ideas on the best ways to manage blood sugars during endurance sports. Soon Paula, with help and encouragement from husband Lew, organized the people she met in races into a not-for-profit organization, calling it the International Diabetic Athletes Association (IDAA). The year was 1985.

Paula sought out people like Edward Horton, MD, and Clifton Bogardus, MD, to serve on the board of directors, as they were well versed in the fields of diabetes and exercise. In addition, Eric Ravussen, PhD, a scientist from the National Institute of Health (NIH) Service, joined the board, and was instrumental in developing it internationally, with subsequent chapters founded in Italy, Greece, the United Kingdom, The Netherlands, Spain, Switzerland and the Dominican Republic.

Today, the revolution and power of diabetes and sports is in full-blown practice among so many people with diabetes. Yes, exercise really is medicine. And if it weren't for our pioneer woman, Paula Harper, perhaps there would not be a Team Type 1 cycling team, professional and Olympic athletes, and other dedicated groups such as Insulindepence, Team Wild, Glucomotive and MADIDEA who encourage and mentor adults and children with diabetes. From the beginning of IDAA, Paula's dream was to encourage people with diabetes to be active, to reach far and live out their dreams. They are runners, bikers, hikers, swimmers, mountaineers, sailors, dancers, paddlers, skaters, basketball, football and baseball players, bodybuilders and fencers. These athletes wear their diabetes proudly, making them role models to inspire others that ... "Hey, we did it, and you can do it too."

How It All Began

Paula was diagnosed with Type 1 diabetes at age twenty-nine, over forty years ago. At the time, she had three young children, ages three months, a year and a half, and three years. Soon after diagnosis, she signed up for a women's sports class, which required running a mile to warm up. That was a brutal wake-up call as to how out of shape she was at the time. Paula became determined to start training and run that one mile.

Her first goal was to run once around a park near her house. That was almost a half-mile. Gradually she increased her distance and gained a little enthusiasm as she found she could meet the goal she set for herself. After a few weeks of running in circles, she took off, aiming towards a more interesting view on the nearby canal banks. Her plan was to run early in the morning before the children woke up and their day started.

Before long Paula was hooked, and running

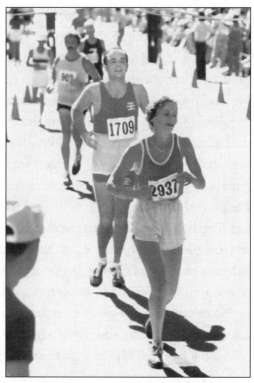

Paula nears another finish line

became a big part of her life. Her husband Lew was supportive and accommodating, which was an important factor—at the time, Paula was in school full time, studying to be an Emergency Room nurse practitioner, and working part time as an ER nurse at the Arizona Health Plant. Three active little ones to care for at home added to her challenge. Taking time for herself was a last priority with such a busy schedule. But Paula found that when she ran it became her own time. Running did great things for her self esteem. Accomplishing goals and the discovery that running also helped with her diabetes management gave her an added sense of pride. Being active on a daily basis lessened her insulin requirements. After a few months Paula began to enter local races, and soon got her speed and endurance up. A year later she felt ready to try a marathon.

The family had a "huddle" about this marathon idea, and decided to make it a special event. So, off they all went to Hawaii in December 1977. What a grand event it turned out to be. Entire families ran together. Young children ran by themselves. There was even a cardiac division for runners who had had heart attacks. An overwhelming feeling of togetherness and compassion marked that whole day. Finishing the race gave Paula a high she had never before experienced. As runners crossed the finish line they were met with big hugs, and seed leis were placed around their necks. A huge picnic and awards ceremony followed afterwards. To top it all, Paula was pleased that she was able to balance food and insulin throughout the run. There were no high-tech meters, CGMs or carb-counting back then, so good guess work ruled the day. And Paula had a strong feeling, almost a dream, about something else that day. How wonderful would it be to have a group of diabetic athletes running together!

Soon after the Hawaiian marathon, Paula's husband Lew got interested in running also, and they started training together. They entered occasional half marathons, with their children often riding bikes alongside as Paula and Lew ran. Next on the Harper family agenda was a family triathlon: second son, Matthew, swam; Lew biked and Paula ran. What great fun to cheer each other on.

Every day of the year in Phoenix, Arizona, is ideal for outdoor exercise, as long as you do it early in the morning. And since Paula was an early riser, she got into a habit of climbing Piestewa Peak (formerly called Squaw Peak), a popular trail—a 1.2 mile hike to the summit. She would leave home in darkness geared up in hiking boots, and carrying a flashlight to test her blood sugar along the way. She hiked this same trail most days of the week for twelve years. Over time it became a social event as Paula got to know other early bird hikers she met along the way. She'd get back home by 6 AM, just as the sun began to pop up in the desert sky and the kids were waking up.

The back side of Camelback Mountain was another favorite hike. Over the years, Paula's enjoyment of hiking took her to the Grand

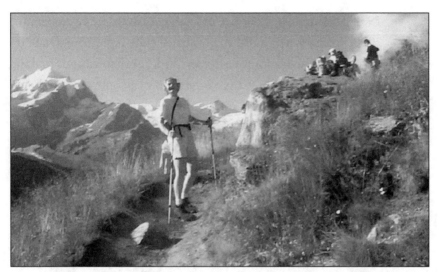

Paula hikes the Swiss Alps, during IDAA conference, Davos

Canyon, which she has traversed rim to rim four times, to several European hiking trails, plus a challenging Swiss Alps trek. When she lived in Nashville, Tennessee, for several years she competed in the annual Country Music Marathon. Paula has completed thirty-five marathon races since that first one in 1977 in Hawaii. She continues to hike the hills around Tucson, Arizona, and has also finished five El Tour de Tucson bike races of one hundred plus mile distances.

Accomplishments as Long as a Marathon

Since founding IDAA/DESA (Diabetes Exercise and Sports Association) nearly thirty years ago, Paula Harper has been fully committed to her belief that sports and exercise are something every person with diabetes should practice daily as a powerful instrument in managing their health. She has received recognition and honors for her work that include:

- 1985: established (along with Clifton Bogardus, MD) the American Diabetes Association Professional Council on Exercise and subsequently served as Chair 1997-1998

- 1992: Distinguished Service in Diabetes Award by Squibb-Novo
- 2000: Josiah Kirby Lilly, Sr. Award by the American Diabetes Association, an honor for a person and/or organizations making outstanding contributions to the lives of people with diabetes, impacting the understanding of diabetes, the ability to improve healthcare and the quality of life for individuals and families
- 2010: Paula and Lew Harper Award created for outstanding young athlete with diabetes.

I have had the honor and privilege to know Paula and serve with her on the board of directors of IDAA/DESA since 1996. She is a true friend to me and a generous spirit, who is concerned and caring enough to motivate and inspire each and every person with diabetes. If it wasn't for Paula Harper, this book might not have been written. So thank you Paula, you are the prime mover for all of us as we go forth in the Sisterhood of Diabetes. ⳾⳽

ARLENE SCHOLER

The Magical Pied Piper
Wears a Backpack

The setting was a hotel in Indianapolis near the National Olympic Training Center at an IDAA (International Diabetes Athletes Association) conference in the spring of 1997. That opening day of the conference had been a long one, and everybody was pretty tired and ready to call it a night. John Walsh—affectionately considered to be the "insulin pump Buddha"—sat in an empty conference room carrying on a conversation with another participant. Somehow, word ignited that John was starting a round table pump talk. Who could resist this opportunity? Within minutes the room filled up with the IDAA crowd, turned out like vagabonds in *I Run On Insulin* T-shirts, mismatched pajamas or sweaty running gear. Soon, the room hummed with excitement, camaraderie and lots of questions for John.

One woman, with an unmistakable New York accent and a tangle of full, thick salt and pepper hair, had a million detailed questions. That was the night I first saw and immediately felt a bond with Arlene Scholer. It wasn't just the New York City accent that made me feel at home with her. It was the energy, the glow that fired within her, that made me want to know more.

"A positive attitude will help you maintain your commitment to a healthier life. Weave your own web of support systems, venture into the world of exertion and give yourself credit for trying!" This is Arlene.

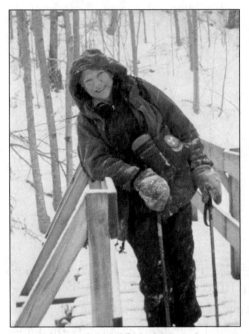

Arlene Scholer

Despite her panoply of worldwide adventures and travels, Arlene still calls home the house where she was born on Long Island. On one of these adventures, camping her way across country with friends in 1964, they wound up partying for several days in San Francisco. One of her group of traveling friends had relatives there who took the band of college girls into their home. While there, Arlene's thirst was without satiation. The official drink of the household was Kool-Aid mixed with pineapple juice, which Arlene guzzled by the gallon. The kids in the family called her "the lady who drank a lot." Arlene attributed her extreme thirst to the socializing she did over the days in San Francisco, visiting the hot spots that the girls had been told about by friends in the know.

Onward to Oregon they ventured. At the outset of the trip she had been the mover and shaker, first one up to do laundry and get breakfast. But by the end she was lethargic and exhausted. While performing her stint at the wheel, a radio commercial caught Arlene's attention. It outlined the symptoms of diabetes, and she counted eight of the ten that applied to her. Not wanting to put a damper on the fun, Arlene kept this to herself and waited, thirstily, until she got back home to go to the doctor. When she told him she thought she had diabetes, he affirmed her diagnosis.

Once the diagnosis became clear, Arlene was put on the standard issue treatment available in 1964 diabetes care, meaning one shot daily of a pretty lousy insulin, injected via glass syringe and a thick 23-gauge steel needle, which she dutifully sharpened with a knife so the "ouch" of the shot wasn't, literally, too much of a pain in the butt. Testing urine by dropping a tablet into a test tube and anxiously hoping it would bubble up blue after two minutes was part of diabetes management back then.

The Hike Begins

Arlene's life as a teacher, her travels with family and friends, biking, downhill and cross country skiing in Vermont and Colorado filled every free weekend and kept her plate full as the years rolled by. Then, things changed for Arlene. As she recalls, "It was August of '77 when a friend and I were traveling through Austria. We took a chairlift up to the top of a mountain and spent the rest of the day hiking down. We were utterly paralyzed for the next three days, but it was my favorite day of the entire vacation and, yes, that's when I fell in love with hiking." A new chapter had begun in her life story.

Since 1977 her love for this sport grew step by step, hike by hike, and continues today. Being outdoors in the fresh air, especially mountain air, in all seasons, had great appeal to Arlene. Once back home from Austria she joined the local chapter of the Adirondack Mountain Club. At first, she was challenged to keep up with all the youngsters who speeded along difficult mountain trails. Loving a challenge, however, Arlene soon graduated from beginner hiker—she was ready for more challenging trails and higher mountains. Camping, backpacking, ice skating and snowshoeing were skills she learned and practiced, and eventually she went on to achieve expert hiking status, sometimes climbing three mountains in a day. Arlene found that the steady even exertion of hiking had the added benefit of keeping good blood sugar control.

What began as an enjoyable vacation day in Austria over thirty years ago led to leading and completing over three hundred hikes in the Catskill Mountains, where winter is her favorite season. Arlene has been active and dedicated in volunteering to maintain trails every fall and

Out of the "Dark Ages" of Diabetes Care

In 1958, a little contraption called **Tes Tape** came on the market—it looked like a carpenter's measuring tape. But instead of a retractable metal ruler, this new gadget dispensed a small roll of indicator paper for testing glucose in the urine. Tes Tape was a minor breakthrough for people with diabetes—you pulled a few inches off the roll and dipped it into drops of urine and waited to see if the strip remained yellow, meaning no sugar, or if it turned a dark green/blue color indicating high sugar. Was it accurate in reading blood glucose levels? No, but it was something. It offered a little encouragement, a little glimmer of light in the dark tunnel of living with diabetes. Tes Tape had some popularity in the early '60's. People even used it to check if there was sugar in soda or wine.

A few years prior, in 1952, a popular **sugar-free soda** named "No-Cal" was invented and introduced, and offered flavors such as root beer, ginger ale and orange. Coca Cola brought out its first sugar-free soda, Tab, about that time. Thinking back, these first attempts of pleasing the diabetic sweet tooth market with effervescent soft drinks were valiant efforts but tasted pretty awful, heavily doused with saccharine and … who knows what other chemicals.

In 1956, **disposable syringes** were patented in New Zealand by a pharmacist/inventor. The American company BD brought the BD Plastipack to market in 1961. It was the same BD that patented the first glass insulin syringes in 1924 (if you were wondering about how long it took to go from glass to disposable). Plastipacks were an instant hit. One could use them and discard them. Or, use them a few times then pitch them. Needles were shorter, sharper and thinner, which equaled less pain. Things were beginning to look up for the diabetes world!

Home Blood Glucose Meter

Urine testing with the archaic methods of old were quickly forgotten when the second greatest discovery—after insulin—came along. The **home**

blood glucose meter really changed the lives and lifestyles of people with diabetes. The first Ames Reflectance Meter, ARM, became available to doctors in 1971 to check patient's blood glucose levels during office visits rather than draw blood and send it out to labs. It was pricey at $495. It basically read, via reflective light, the blood glucose level of a Dextro-stick and gave it a number. "**Dextro-sticks**" and "**Clini-sticks**" (1963–65) were litmus indicator paper strips that were a step up from TesTape since they had the capacity to read blood instead of urine, thus giving a more accurate account of real blood glucose. Scientists discovered how to pinpoint the readings even further with the advent of the bg meter.

The home blood glucose monitor travelled from the doctor's office into the patients' homes with the help of a diabetic patient named Richard Bernstein. An engineer at the time, Richard questioned his doctor about using this meter on his own to check his blood sugar. It came down the corporate pike that a prescription was necessary to insure that the doctor would be responsible for training the patient to use the meter correctly. Engineer Bernstein's wife happened to be a doctor. She wrote the prescription and, in time, after years of trying to convince the diabetes community that the meter *really worked*, Bernstein himself decided that, in order to get his case studies of diabetes and meters recognized, he would need the authority of a doctor full time! And so, at age forty-seven, he went to medical school. Today Dr. Richard Bernstein remains an active endocrinologist specializing in diabetes care. He has written several books on the subject.

The Insulin Pump

In the early '70s the first **insulin pump** came on the market as an obtuse backpack contraption that few people knew about or were interested in using when they saw what it looked liked and what it entailed.

Picture a microwave oven! You know its approximate size. Now picture an insulin pump. You know its size as well. It might be a little difficult to imagine that, in the early 1970s, insulin pumps were the size of microwaves. They were called **biostaters**. Their primary use was to treat diabetic ketoacidosis (DKA) in hospitals. A California doctor, Arnold Kadish, is credited with inventing the first insulin pump in the early 1960s. In the 1970s other scientists, notably Dean Kamen, came up the notion of letting diabetes patients regulate their own insulin pumps based on results from their glucose meters. The idea came from portable pumps used by cancer patients to infuse chemotherapy drugs. More ideas began to percolate in research labs. The size of pumps shrunk to sixteen-ounce backpack types, with external syringes. From there, scientists and inventors went to work on further minimizing and improving the subcutaneous insulin infusion delivery system. The first published papers came out of Guy's Hospital, London, from a group of research doctors that included Dr. J. C. Pickup.

Even though the first pumps were unreliable, bulky and cumbersome, in order to be accepted as a candidate for pump use one had to undergo psychological testing, do a one-week stint in the hospital, and sign "in blood" (not literally) that she or he would faithfully take on the responsibility to do regular blood-glucose monitoring.

The year was 1983 when, at an American Diabetes Association conference, the first user-friendly FDA-approved insulin pump was unveiled by Minimed. Minimed in the U.S. and Disetronic (Swiss) in Europe had the market cornered up until the 1990s when it became clear through studies that insulin pump therapy with its tight control not only showed lower HbA1c results but allowed a more flexible lifestyle for the user. Other companies began manufacturing insulin pumps and today the climate remains fertile and competitive.

New improved features, better accuracy and durability are the results of such competition. The idea of a **continuous glucose monitoring system** started brewing in 1962 and reached the marketplace in 1999. Now we see the merging of CGMs and pumps as they integrate on their way to a closed loop system which will test glucose levels and deliver insulin all in one neat little package.

Yes, we still wake up every morning with diabetes as our partner. And yes, we still base our lifestyle on healthy eating and daily exercise and yes, it makes us strong and vibrant if we do this with a positive attitude. Like any relationship, there are good days and rough ones, but we still greet each new day with possibilities, a healthy lifestyle, ever-refined technology and marvelous dreams. Thank God for those intrepid pioneers who led the way for us. ⊱⊰

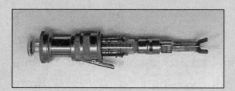

Busher's Automatic Injector used in the 1950s

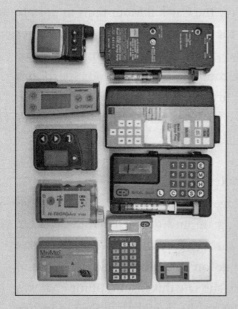

Old pumps (from upper left corner: Autosyringe AS-6C, Autosyringe AS6MP, CPI/ Lilly 9100, Minimed 502, CPI/ Lilly 9200, Minimed 504-S, Disetronic H-TRONplus V100, Anumas R1000, Disetronic D-TRON, and Animas IR-1200)
Photo credit John Walsh

spring in her beloved mountains. Teaching snowshoeing for twenty-five years in those mountains brought as much joy and fun for her as it did for students.

There have been other hikes on other mountains through the years. Arlene summited forty-six peaks in the Adirondacks, forty-two peaks in New Hampshire, and an assortment of glorious peaks in the Rocky Mountains. One of Arlene's brothers lives at 6,200 foot elevation in the majestic Rockies, and when Arlene visits, the entire family enjoys hikes in that neighborhood.

Always the Teacher

For fifteen years Arlene co-taught backpacking and started a group called the Empowerment Series, which encouraged new hikers from her home base on Long Island to try the Catskill Mountains in upstate New York. The groups started in the fall, with each hike being farther and higher, and by winter Arlene taught them one of the joys and fun of winter hiking—snowshoeing. The combination of outdoor sports and her natural inclination as teacher, organizer and leader have all woven together for good health and good diabetes care. I think of Arlene as "magical pied piper who wears a backpack."

Exercising an Option with Diabetes

The year was 1980. Life was fast paced as usual. But Arlene's blood sugars were busy too, wildly riding up and down the roller coaster. Those after-breakfast highs were causing havoc with control. An aggressive doctor suggested that Arlene go on something called an "insulin pump" to solve the problem. When she saw this insulin pump that was supposed to help regulate blood sugars, she thought it looked more like a WW II walkie-talkie than a medical device. She was not very keen on the idea, but agreed that if her blood glucose levels were not better off in the summer, she would go into the hospital for a week at Thanksgiving to try this new fangled insulin pump.

The blood sugars did not really improve much and so, living up to the one week commitment she made to her doctor, Arlene agreed to go into the hospital, giving up skiing, hiking and a big family Thanksgiving celebration. The good news was that the design and size of the pump had improved slightly over the one she had first seen. The new model was only about nine inches long and actually had a cover. The next hurdle to jump was finding a hospital in her area that would admit a diabetic patient about to go on an insulin pump. On the fourth try they found one willing to take on the challenge.

It's almost hard to imagine those first pumps since today even a two-inch by three-inch pump with tubing is practically archaic. Tubeless pumps with remote readers and continuous glucose monitors are commonplace today. Soon a closed loop system that tests and delivers insulin all in one neat little package, something that once seemed futuristic, will be arriving at our doorstep. Pump technology certainly has progressed since those pioneer days thirty long years ago.

Crossroads and Challenges

Even though one follows the guidelines and plays according to the rules diabetes puts forward, pop-ups, crossroads and detour signs can appear. Arlene, intrepid soul that she is, has faced several snags along the pathway of trying to adhere to excellent diabetes management. There was the broken hip from an ice skating fall, knee replacement surgeries due to years of overuse, diabetic neuropathy and the loss of vision in one eye. Despite these challenges, Arlene attributes diabetes for her state of general good health. Because of diabetes she has pursued physical exercise as a means of keeping blood sugars in line. For her it's all about being outdoors and moving. Her philosophy of "I'd rather pull weeds than be indoors" has inspired her to do all her own yard work including raking leaves, shoveling snow, transplanting bushes and shrubs, landscaping, cleaning gutters and other home maintenance chores.

Strong family ties are a staple in Arlene's life. Growing up in a working-class family, Arlene's loving parents always stressed the importance of receiving the best possible education. Arlene became a teacher; one brother is a retired mechanical engineer who designed power plants; her other brother received two PhDs in chemistry and taught at Cornell. Their parents, both deceased now, would certainly have swelled with pride in their children.

Arlene never married and has no pets, which means she is the lucky one who gets to travel to Colorado and Chincoteague, Maryland, to visit and spend time with family members. Speaking of Chincoteague, a couple of years ago I was lucky enough to make it down there to one of her famous "Chincoteague and Assauteague Wild Pony Weekends." What fun! Arlene the great organizer set forth a weekend of cycling, walking, birding, swimming in the Atlantic, observing herds of wild ponies, kayaking, dining and general fun and camaraderie for a group of fellow DESA members. We stayed in her brother's house and a neighboring house, both on a beautiful lake, for a spectacular September weekend.

A Good Match

Over twenty years ago a friend showed Arlene a newspaper article on IDAA (International Diabetes Athletes Association), now known as DESA (Diabetes Exercise and Sports Association). She tracked down Paula Harper, IDAA founder and president, and offered to write an article entitled "Exercise Your Options" which covered the demands of pump therapy when hiking and camping in all seasons. The article talked about rechargeable batteries and the fun of camping at minus twenty-five degrees. It was written in 1988 and still holds much validity and smart suggestions.

Arlene and IDAA/DESA was a perfect match. In addition to valuing the information and education at national conferences, she cherished the social interaction with other diabetic athletes. In the 1990s Arlene planned two extended weekends of hiking, biking and paddling in beautiful Lake Placid, New York, for the DESA membership. There were thirty attendees each weekend from around the U.S., Canada and Australia. Today a core group from Lake Placid maintains a friendship and shared adventures. They have hiked the Catskill Mountains, kayaked waterways from the Florida Keys to northern Florida to North Carolina to Maryland. Whenever there is a DESA conference they plan their adventures around it by arriving early to renew friendships. They have walked and hiked and visited local breweries and fine restaurants from Vancouver, B.C. to Westchester, Pennsylvania.

Better Health

Arlene attributes involvement with DESA for finding health professionals from whom she has learned so much about fine-tuning her diabetes management. In 1997, Gary Scheiner, CDE and DESA friend, taught Arlene how to count carbohydrates, which allows her "permission" to indulge in an occasional dish of sherbet—although if she had the freedom to do so, she'd eat ice cream for breakfast, lunch and dinner every day. Perhaps it comes from her natural teacher instinct that Arlene has kept HbA1c (Glycosolated Hemoglobin blood test, which reflects blood glucose average for the previous two-three months) records since 1979. [By the way, Arlene's average out to 5.9, which is practically a non-diabetic number. Wow!] Being an active person for so many years has kept her in shape and fit to continue to pursue at least an hour of exercise each morning plus afternoon destination walks and bike rides.

I asked Arlene about how she sees her long life with diabetes as a partner and she told me:

When I started hiking in '77 I asked my doctor for some advice. He replied: "What can I tell you? Most of my patients are couch potatoes." Learning to independently manage my diabetes with my insulin pump has given me a sense of pride. I have been on pump therapy since 1980, and the first fifteen years were a roll of

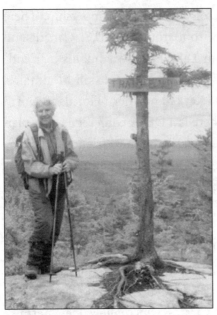

Arlene at the top of the mountain

the dice as I learned from my own mistakes. Help from John Walsh and Gary Scheiner in the nineties has surely helped.

As for seeing a cure for diabetes:

I have heard that promise since 1964. I'm just grateful for the pump and glucose meters, and continuous glucose monitors that make my personal control so much easier. I have always been aggressive about my diabetes control. Careful meal planning and calculated insulin boluses reward me with good health and multiple snacks, on top of hearty meals of eighty to one-hundred carbohydrate grams.

I have told friends that if they were to walk into a gathering of diabetics at a DESA conference, they'd think they were in a room with healthy athletes who have accomplished super goals. Being as active as I can be at age seventy, I hope I can project a YES I CAN attitude to the average person who is accustomed to seeing sedentary, non-exercising diabetics.

Arlene Scholer has been a great inspiration to me, as someone who has lived with Type 1 diabetes since 1962. More than this, she embodies what the Sisterhood of Diabetes is all about: perseverance, positive attitude, doing one's best, a sense of adventure and enthusiasm for life. If you have been lucky enough to meet this motivating, powerhouse pied piper wearing a backpack, you know what I mean!   🦋

PATRICIA RUHE KEHS

Living the Good Life with Diabetes at 94+

Pat Kehs was diagnosed with Type 2 diabetes when she was eighty-three years old. She immediately learned all she could about treatment and possible consequences of Type 2 diabetes from her long-time family doctors, Dennis McGorry Sr. and Jr., and signed up for a diabetes education course. With a few minor adjustments, her life would not change much. She was determined to control this surprise visitor to her long and productive life by utilizing her healthy diet and daily exercise. Pat told me: "Diabetes made me step up my walking and exercise program. I think I get exercise from gardening also, all that up and down, bending and reaching. That's exercise!"

There is always something going on in Pat's life. She keeps busy socially with friends, and her two devoted daughters,

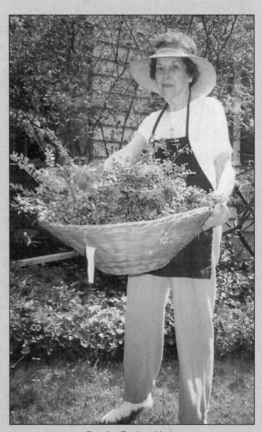

Paula Ruhe Kehs

Katrina and Deidre, keep Pat involved with all the good things life has to offer. Her only complaint is dealing with problems that naturally occur in a ninety-plus-year-old body. But staying active and interested in life makes those aches and pains a lot easier to take.

Reading the *New York Times* from cover to cover every day as well as the *New Yorker Magazine* keeps her up to the minute on everything that's going on in the world. She clips and sends articles of interest to friends of all ages who live all over the country. Long conversational letters always accompany the articles, and there are usually a few pressed flowers in the envelopes as well.

End of summer is apple time in Allentown, Pennsylvania. There is a big old grafted apple tree in the Kehs backyard. Every year it hangs heavy with half red stripe and half greening apples. This is the signal for Pat to get out the Foley food mill that belonged to her mother and get to work, peeling cutting up and milling the apples to make the most delicious applesauce in Eastern Pennsylvania. She winds up giving most of the applesauce away to people who just happen to stop by every year during apple season. The process of making the applesauce has always been both a joy and a lesson in persistence and discipline.

Self discipline has inspired Pat to get all the things she has wanted in life. This quality has really helped her deal with diabetes. She hopes a cure will find its way to everyone who lives with diabetes. In the meantime she's eating fresh and healthy food from her vegetable garden, taking a daily walk, doing exercises at home and enjoying and living her life with a smile on her face and twinkle in her beautiful eyes. Pat Ruhe Kehs is certainly an inspiration to all the sisters who together, from all walks of life and all ages, make up the magic and power of the Sisterhood of Diabetes. ❧

CHAPTER 2

The Pros

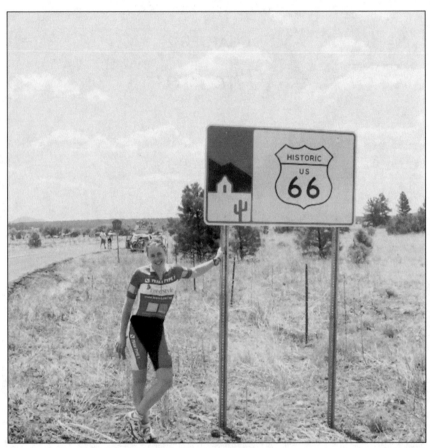

Monique Hanley

MONIQUE HANLEY

Spins Wheels and Inspiration

M onique Hanley grew up on the dairy farm where her parents still live in a hamlet called Yarragon (population 600) in Warragul, Victoria, Australia, about sixty miles east of Melbourne. Translated from its local Aboriginal roots, Yarragon means "Dingo" or wild dog." Usual visitors to the family farm include wombats, cockatoos, kookaburras, snakes and kangaroos. Truth is, time stands still in this verdant, lush splendid corner of the world.

An annual event called the Great Victorian Bike Ride takes place there, and stretches out over nine days. One year, Monique's mother, an avid recreational cyclist, completed the ride with Monique's oldest brother. The other kids in the family loved hearing the stories of this great adventure, and naturally they all wanted to take part in it. And so a family rule was firmly established. When each of the other three siblings turned fourteen, they would ride the Great Vic. For Monique, it was a fantastic experience that firmly set a love of cycling in her heart.

Monique was a jock from the get-go in a sports crazy country. She participated in Little Athletics, netball, swimming and tennis, and achieved first-place wins every year though high school in cross country. While still in elementary school, Monique was chosen to represent her district in a cricket clinic at the Melbourne Cricket Ground, which holds 100,000 people. But, gradually, basketball became her one true love. She was a terrific player who relished defensive moves, knowing what the offense was going to do before they knew it themselves, and loved setting up plays for her team to score. Monique played all through her high school and university years. In fact, her whole life was basketball.

At nineteen, Monique was playing basketball at the second highest level in Australia, just under the women's national basketball league. It was at the close of pre-season training when Monique was diagnosed with Type 1 diabetes. As she told me:

I had all the symptoms: thirst, fatigue, dry skin, polyuria, blurry vision. These annoyances were beginning to affect my game. It was time to go to the doctor to see if there was something wrong. When it was officially confirmed that I had diabetes, I had three things I wanted to make clear with the doctor straight away before any more details of this condition were to be disclosed. My breathing stopped when I thought of the first issue. "I play basketball," I exploded at the doctor in a way of challenging him to tell me I couldn't do it, but he was smart enough to tell me I could continue to play. My next point was an overseas student trip to study for a semester at Ryerson Polytechnic University in Toronto, Canada. Again a wave of panic set in at the thought of having to cancel the trip. When he informed me that people with diabetes can travel, I began to breathe again. Whew! My thoughts next turned to an upcoming university social gathering where I had already paid a huge amount of my miniscule income towards a ticket. The precious ticket also included an evening's worth of drinks. I blurted "and I drink alcohol." Drinking age is eighteen in Australia. The doc explained that drinking alcohol is certainly possible with a few precautions and that I would soon learn all about them in the coming weeks. After that I didn't care what they said or did. In my mind, life could still go on.

A Love Lost

One week after her diagnosis, Monique set a top five best record for team assists which still stands at the Dandenong Rangers basketball team. Four months later she was off to Toronto to study at Ryerson Polytechnic University. As soon as she got herself settled, she immediately found her way to the gym to play a little pick-up basketball. Her hard working, tough, honest and very defensive Aussie style of playing the game attracted the attention of the coaches, and she was quickly signed onto the varsity team where she became a stunning asset.

After finishing her degree in economics and strategic planning, Monique worked for economic consulting firms in Canada and Australia for five years. From there she advanced to a job with the State Government of Victoria. But the change in lifestyle—working, training full time, playing games and tournaments and managing diabetes—brought her an unexpected amount of stress. Monique stopped enjoying the sport she had loved so much. Her life was scattered in too many directions and so she decided it was time to concentrate on work and managing her diabetes. Understandably, leaving basketball was a tough decision, and the only way for her to do it was to make a quick break. She finished out the season and then, cold turkey, walked off the court and never looked back.

Shifting Gears

When Monique stopped playing basketball she was unable to control her diabetes and maintain a slender muscular body. Her endocrinologist pointed out that it would be necessary to exercise daily to keep her diabetes and weight well managed. Applying her sense of discipline and determination to succeed, Monique found the answer.

Fortunately, she was living in Melbourne's inner city at this time, where it was much easier to get around on a bike. Recalling the days of family adventures riding the Great Vic, Monique thought that biking could serve as both exercise and transportation. When she purchased her new bike, a love affair began to blossom.

Monique remembered how she and her brother glued themselves to the television for the Tour de France every year, and how she stuck pictures of five-time winner, Miguel Indurain, on all her school books. Distance cycling became Monique's new pursuit in 2000.

Her first challenge was a one-day, 130-mile event. Although on the edge of extreme nervousness about managing her diabetes for this distance, she wound up coming to the aid of her struggling non-diabetic partner, helping him cross the finish line. This success motivated her to keep riding and building her skills for another year. In 2002, she cycled 7,800 km across Canada in sixty-six days, fortifying her strength and endurance and gaining a large dose of confidence in managing diabetes. By 2003, she decided she was ready to follow the Tour de France route ... solo ... armed with a few months of French conversation lessons, her trusty steel-framed road bike (dubbed "Harry") and a small rear-pack containing a sleeping bag, mat and a change of clothes. She wore a lightweight backpack stuffed with a one person tent, while hanging off the handlebars another small pack held her passport, language guide, maps and one month's supply of insulin and diabetes testing equipment. While the professional riders covered 3,400 km over three weeks, Monique completed 2,600 km on her own, battling navigational issues, language barriers and the daily trial of finding somewhere safe to stay for the night.

I had planned this trip to be on the cheap, which was why I brought a tent with me. But my first day riding out of Paris took so long that I realized I needed to amend my plans as I went. Also, my budget accommodation plan to camp by the side of the road seemed reasonable when I was in Australia. However when faced with the real world of a non-English speaking countryside, I could not put myself in a vulnerable position. I was so scared at the thought of it that on my first day I just kept riding until it was almost dark. Finally a solution came to mind.

*I noticed a sign for a "Gite," a rural bed and breakfast estab-
lishment. I rode into the farmyard of this property and with my
limited language skills negotiated to camp in their backyard. Not
only did I feel somewhat safer, I also had access to a shower after
a long day of riding. The proprietors were so shocked by my crazi-
ness that they didn't charge me and even fed me breakfast in the
morning. From that day, my new budget-accommodation-plan
was set around this scenario. Along with it, I had the benefit of
meeting locals which I would never have had the chance to do if I
was on the side of the road.*

Monique witnessed eleven live stages of the Tour de France and
rode on much of the course route, including the famous climbs of
Alpe D'Huez and the Col du Tourmalet (*http://en.wikipedia.org/wiki/
Col_du_Tourmalet*).You can read about her amazing trip on the Tour at
www.moniquehanley.com.

Following this epic adventure, Monique sought a next challenge.
Attending track cycling at the local velodrome was always a great family
pastime, highlighted by a family trip to Sydney for the 2000 Olympics.
But the 2004 World Track Championships in Melbourne became the
turning point for Monique. Here she witnessed Australian Katie Mactier
go neck to neck with New Zealand's Sarah Ulmer in the individual-
pursuit track-cycling final. That same year, watching on TV the Athens
2004 Olympics—in which Australia won numerous gold medals in
track cycling—"sealed my fate that I would take up this sport somehow,
some way."

For Monique, track racing in general was of benefit for two main
reasons: she possessed a natural endurance sprint, well suited to the
longer track distances, and she had plenty of time to train hard and test
her blood glucose levels between efforts. The physical intensity of the
training—consisting of short intense efforts with longer recovery time,
gave her the opportunity to test blood glucose levels between efforts,

allowing for better management of her diabetes. Compared to long days out in the road bike, clocking up mile after mile without any knowledge of what was happening to her blood sugar, this seemed ideal.

Track racing allows for close, high intensity racing, which presented a whole new challenge for an athlete with diabetes, and for the first time Monique encountered problems with the impact of adrenaline. The huge rush from racing shocked her body into releasing glucose from her liver and spiked her blood glucose, which then remained elevated for hours. When the liver releases stored glucose, the blood glucose levels raise accordingly. It becomes a tricky situation to get those high bg numbers back into a normal range. This is compounded when an athlete is performing at high stress levels. Frequent monitoring or checking the levels, along with careful dosing of insulin to bring the levels back to a relatively normal range, must be given attention. At high levels of competition, an athlete tries to keep blood sugar numbers as even as possible since fluctuations can not only weaken performance but make the athlete feel quite ill.

Monique also discovered criterium racing—a short circuit, often with a number of corners that required explosive acceleration, solid bike handling skills, and a steel resolve to turn corners without applying any brakes. Races consist of repeating the circuit multiple times for about one hour. This exciting format suited her body type and she steadily improved in it.

Insulin Injected Engines

Monique's next challenge was finding others with diabetes to train and ride with. This inspired her to bellow out across Victoria for active Type 1s to unite for the sake of sports, and led to the creation of HypoActive, *www. hypoactive.org*. The mission of this organization is to promote, encourage and teach active and athletic lifestyles for Type 1 diabetics. Its tag line, which appears on their riding jerseys, is "Insulin Injected Engines." The organization has grown steadily and broadened its scope of activities since Monique co-founded it in 2004. HypoActive not only organizes team sports but also mentors new athletes of all ages and levels of exercise.

Once Monique began distance and track cycling there was no stopping this tough young woman. She competed in races all around Australia and won several State Championships. People in the international track and criterium cycling circuit were taking notice that Monique was a winning force. In 2007, she placed third in the Australian National Track Championships. Around that time Monique discovered a U.S. based cycling team for people with Type 1 diabetes called "Team Type 1." For her it seemed a match made in heaven. She excitedly contacted the founders, Phil Southerland and Joe Eldridge, who politely declined her initial enthusiastic approach. However, Monique's strong performances continued and, after being the dominant Victorian rider across the 2006/7 season, she was invited to join Team Type 1 in the 2007 Race Across America (RAAM) team. RAAM consists of racing 3,500 miles across the U.S. from west coast to east coast. It is a non-stop endurance event of epic proportions.

The Ride
Put yourself on a virtual bicycle as you read about some of the things the RAAM team experienced during the 3,500 mile adventure.

- 100,000 ft. of climbing
- Three massive mountain passes
- The unforgiving heat and treacherous conditions through Monument Valley
- The long climbs of Colorado with elevation factor and lack of oxygen
- The steep climbs of Virginia
- The short sharp ups and downs through the Ozarks
- The long, drawn out prairies across Kansas
- The twists and turns through Lancaster County, Pennsylvania
- Snow in Colorado

- Floods in the mid-west
- A team of nineteen support crew
- A team of eight riders—all with Type 1 diabetes, five "first time" riders and three one-year veterans
- A great big target on their backs as defending champions
- Nausea and nosebleeds from the elevations in Arizona, Utah and Colorado and later simply nausea from eating too much cycling-specific food products
- Head winds, cross winds and severe thunderstorms

In 2006, Team Type 1 had finished an agonizing second. They returned in 2007 determined to make that step to the top of the podium and recruited accordingly. Monique's position was indeed unique on the team—seven guys and her. Being a firecracker cyclist with a snappy twist of Aussie wit made it all work. TT1 crossed the finish line of the 3,500 mile race in a victorious record breaking 5 days, 15 hours, 43 minutes, averaging 22.54 mph.

There was reason to celebrate on many fronts that year. The first cycling team consisting of all Type 1 diabetic athletes had pedaled their way to victory from Oceanside, California to Atlantic City, New Jersey, and this triumphant moment marked a collective turning point, shattering the long-held myth that people with diabetes could and should not hope to be endurance athletes. We all knew we could do anything we set our hearts on, but now, in prime time, the entire world could witness it and blink their eyes.

RAAM Keeps Riding

In 2008 the Norwegians beat out TT1 but TT1 came back to shatter their 2007 win and break new records in 2009 and again in 2010. To defend their title every year, they needed to be on top of their diabetes game, making sure that glucose levels are in the zone throughout the race. They used the Freestyle Navigator continuous glucose monitoring system to assist in tracking blood sugar levels but plenty of testing and other management tools are used as well. Ideally, massive high blood sugars and bad low blood sugars can be warded off, but living with diabetes one knows that it doesn't take much for these things to happen. We can only do our best.

One of the Girls

Monique's career as a professional track cyclist and strong advocate of living an active diabetes lifestyle has inspired many, and she takes her position as a role model seriously. In 2007, at the Friends For Life, Children With Diabetes conference in Orlando, Florida, she told me that she felt unsure of herself speaking to and trying to inspire such a large group of kids. She wanted to excite them, and when she posed the question, "Who wants to ride with me to beat out the boys?" the girls cheered and waved their arms wildly in the air. She had captured her audience and now she would be able to motivate them.

I got to know Monique at the end of the 2007 DESA Colorado Springs conference. I was standing waiting for a taxi to the airport when Monique walked by. After a minute of chit chat she, very matter-of-factly, insisted that I check my blood sugar. Naturally, I resisted, but she wouldn't hear of it. I acquiesced and tested. It was 58. She watched while I ate a few candies, thanked her, and wished her well with her upcoming races. "I'm not going anywhere until your blood sugar is up past 70," she said. When I told her the cab would be there any second, she responded by saying she would go to the airport with me if needed. In a few minutes my blood sugar jumped up to 72 and all turned out fine. What caring and kindness this twenty-nine-year-old superstar had shown to me, a fellow diabetic sister. Monique Hanley became part of the inspiration to write this book.

Bumpy Road Ahead

On May 30, 2009, in the first ten minutes of the Tulsa Tough race (Oklahoma), at the top of her brilliant career as a professional athlete, Monique was riding near the wall with no place to move when a rider slid across in front of her. Next thing, Monique was off her bike and airborne. When she landed, she had spinous process fractures of thoracic 2, 3, 4, and 5 vertebrae. In other words, a broken back, along with a separation of the acromioclavicular (AC) joint in her shoulder.

After a stay in a U.S. hospital, Monique returned home to Australia for the surgery. Due to hospital policy, her Omnipod insulin pump had to be removed until post surgery, and consequently her blood sugars raged for days after the operation. An active life of flying fast and furious on a bicycle had abruptly come to an accidental full stop.

Monique's healing process was devastating for her. She struggled with the "why and how and what for" demons for long days and nights. But, being an intrepid soul, she soon got to work again with HypoActive projects. She exercised by walking her dog, a pretty boring sport for a speed demon like Monique. Yet family and friends were always there to encourage her.

After a frustrating six months of recovery, Monique was back on her bike and starting to race again. She returned to the U.S. in 2010 to signal her return to pro-level racing. However, in the week before departing Australia she discovered a wonderful surprise—she was pregnant.

A New Challenge and an Old Challenge
A quick check with her doctor indicated that she could race while visiting the U.S, provided she did not compete in hot conditions. Nevertheless, she found untimely nausea to coincide with intense physical outputs, and further medical advice confirmed her fears: racing while pregnant was simply not possible. Despite this, she continued to follow her husband as an observer on their tour of the U.S. racing circuit.

Returning to Tulsa, Oklahoma, and the scene of the horrific crash of 2009, Monique determined to erase the lingering memory of that disastrous race in her own way. Armed with (one) doctor's cautious okay to race, and cognizant of her own physical limitations from the new life growing inside her, she fronted up to the start line. Adrenaline pumped ... and so did the temperature—it was 100 degrees F, but Monique knew she had to overcome the fear and the nightmares of the past twelve months and get around the circuit safely.

She couldn't be in better company to re-visit the scene of so much pain. One lap was completed and a smile burst open on her face. She was okay. By lap three she rounded the last corner to lead the field through the start/finish line and across the exact spot in the course where she had crashed. What a feeling! Conscious to avoid over-heating, she then pulled out of the race, milestone accomplished, and embraced husband Ewin.

One of her dreams was always to have children. Monique gave birth to Amelie in January 2010, and at the time of this writing is pregnant with her second child.

Monique wrote something recently that concluded, "Until we meet again, may the roads be well paved, clear of traffic, the wind at your back and may your glucose levels be 99."

Same to you, unique Monique Hanley, a true diabetes hero, a sister and role model for all. Check out updates at: *www.moniquehanley.com*

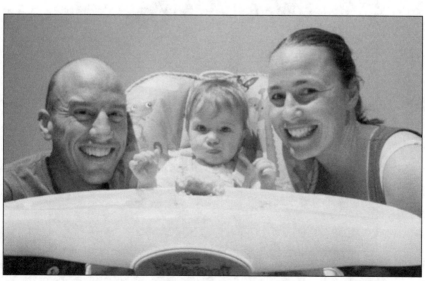

Ewin and Monique celebrate baby Amelie

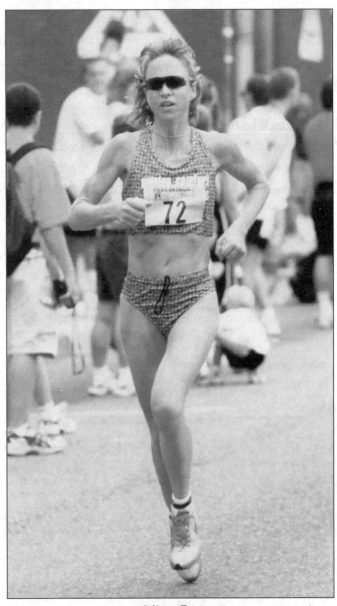

Missy Foy

Leader of the Pack

M issy Foy … Missy Foy … Missy Foy, the name turns heads in elite running circles just as it does in the active, athletic diabetes community. Her accomplishments and lists of "firsts" run deep, and carry weight and substance.

- Started racing in 1996
- Signed onto a national women's racing team in 1999
- Was a member of USATF Olympic Development program for two years
- Voted North Carolina's Runner of the Year 1997 and 1998
- Awarded the 1999 LifeScan Athletic Achievement Award
- In 1999, first athlete with diabetes to qualify for the 2000 Olympic Marathon Trials
- In 2005, broke into the ultra marathon running scene with a record breaking (by 20 minutes) performance in the challenging Umstead Endurance Run's 50-mile trail race
- 2007, on the podium with a silver medal in the U.S. 50-Mile National Championships

First Impressions

To be in Missy's presence is electrifying. If you put Missy in competition with a deer running in the forest, my bet would be on Missy. I have been around her in a peripheral way, meeting at various CWD (Children With Diabetes) and DESA (Diabetes Exercise and Sports Association) conferences over the years. But, I never really knew her wit and wisdom, her agility in dealing with people from all walks, her gritty determination, fanned with an appropriately sweet southern drawl, her warmth and kindness and her capacity to make difficult things seem breezy. Missy Foy is swift footed and thoughtful as she paces herself along life's highways and byways, knowing how to turn at crossroads, coast down hills and relax when the moment allows.

One chilly weekend in winter 2012, Missy called to tell me she would be coming up to New York City to host a bridal shower for Heidi, her "kid sister" who really wasn't a sister but a close friend and running protégé. We made a plan to meet and I offered to take her around town to pick up things she needed for the shower. I told her she could hop a taxi to our meeting spot, but being the adventurer that she is, Missy navigated her way through the labyrinth of the NYC subway system. It was unusually bitter and windy

Missy's First Steps

As you know, it's an odd story how I got started running at age twenty-eight. I had left grad school and was working in medical research. My husband Bob was running two to three miles twice a week because he had to stay in shape for the Army Reserves. Plus, there were several people where I worked who would go running a few times a week in the afternoon. So, I had been thinking about running when one day at work I had lower abdominal pain, ended up in the emergency room and had my appendix out by that night. The appendectomy for some reason made me feel really old and frail so I turned my prior thoughts about running into action. I went over to the track at Duke and wanted to be able to run two miles without stopping. The first time I could barely make a mile. I was persistent and kept going back though, and met Wade who had experienced a serious heart attack the prior year. He was introduced to running through a cardiac rehab program at Duke and never looked back. Wade and I became good friends and ended up running road races together. It actually took me a couple years before I realized I wasn't frail and had potential to run well. At first it was just something that made me feel empowered because I felt fit and strong. Eventually it became a lifestyle change and all the insecure feelings were put to rest.

So, that's the story of how and why I started running. I wasn't a high school or college phenom or anything even close. I trained smart and was very patient, which is how I reached my potential.

that day as we crisscrossed our way uptown, downtown and cross-town to buy wine, chocolates, coffee and gifts. Five hours later, laden down with shopping bags and boxes, hungry and exhausted, we finally sat down to kick back and chitchat.

What Makes Missy Run?

Being the first girl born into her father's family in fifty years, Missy spent most of her youth surrounded by boys and brothers. There was only one other girl in her neighborhood and she was a tomboy too, just like Missy. When she was seven, all Missy wanted for Christmas was a New York Jets football uniform. She wore her Jets uniform until threadbare, and when it no longer fit, she turned to basketball. Longing to be a power forward, Missy discovered she was just too small. Undeterred, she went on to become a power swimmer.

Missy always had a strong streak of competition and determination. Even as a little girl during family walks at night in summertime, she always tried to make her shadow lead everybody else's.

The question of Type 1 diabetes and standing up to challenges is a classic debate we all have. Does diabetes spawn competitiveness and the urge to prove that we really can do anything "normal" non-diabetics can do and maybe even do it better? Or, is it that the precision and discipline of diabetes makes competition a comfortable milieu and natural habitat?

Missy's sense of competitiveness was a part of who she was long before diabetes knocked at the door. From competing over the length of her shadow as a little girl, she continued to excel throughout her school years where she was always at the top of her class, in the ninety-nine percentile of academic rankings. But, at a certain point in eighth grade she became weary of being a "brainiac" and "geek" and started high school feeling uncomfortable and self-conscious. Missy then withdrew socially, although she maintained her academic status. It was in college where she fully regained her self esteem and felt proud to be a smart and competent young woman. Missy completed her Ph.D. in the history of medicine at the University of North Carolina.

On July 26, 2007 the *New York Times* reported: "Diabetic and Determined. When Missy Foy was diagnosed with type 1 diabetes some 12 years ago, in her own words, "I totally freaked out. I cried for days."

She was launching a career into elite running circles.

Enter Diabetes

When Missy was first diagnosed with Type 1 in 1997 at age thirty-three, she was a dedicated competitive runner who had just qualified for the U.S. Half Marathon National Championships. It was the second time she had qualified for a national championship race. On Wednesday before the Saturday race, she became violently ill with a recurrence of food poisoning that had been lingering for days. In the wee hours of Sunday morning, August 24 to be exact, Missy, feeling absolutely miserable, lay in bed in an emergency room at the local hospital. The attending physician and a resident walked over to her bed and told her that in addition to a case of *campylobacter* (a strain of food poisoning) she had a very high blood sugar which indicated Type 1 diabetes. Missy's spirits sunk to the ground. She believed that any prospects of a professional running career were now fried.

The Learning Process Begins

Because it's not in Missy's intrepid nature to give up on things, she determined to weave diabetes and running together to make it possible for her to follow her dream of being a professional runner. When I asked Missy about her attitude towards having diabetes she said,

> *I actually hate having diabetes. I hate the scheduling, the routine, the constant checking that goes on in the back of my mind. I don't like needles and have never learned to jab one on in. But I'm not going to sit around and cry about it. It just is what it is and I can't change it. There are worse things to have to live with. Diabetes is manageable. It's not fun or exciting but it's manageable and that's the attitude I keep … most days!*

The rocky road to understanding how to match diabetes, training and racing was one huge trial and error lesson. At first, when her blood sugar would plummet during and after running, she thought her fitness level had suddenly become affected by diabetes and that she needed to train harder. Over the first year of dealing with the many realities and subtleties of living with diabetes, Missy learned how her body worked. Most of all, she now understood how to pursue a competitive running career. She knew she could not run without insulin on board. She had tried that and it simply did not work. Blood sugars torpedoed. So she analyzed and tested which foods and quick carb products worked best for her nutritional needs, and how well she tolerated them. She experimented with sites and times of insulin injections, as well as different insulin and insulin pumps. She kept flawless records of every training session. It was like going to a job or school everyday … working hard to achieve a goal and, once everything about it had been accomplished with flying colors, going on to the next challenge. Each step of the way was crafted with precision, discipline, research, tedious repetition, planning and more planning. After about a year of this, Missy felt comfortable and confident that she could surge ahead and set achievable racing goals.

Marathon Missy

In December of 1998 Missy completed her first marathon in 3:00:45. She remembers the experience as being grueling, and feeling nauseous throughout the race. Undaunted, she was determined to do better. Three months later she ran her second marathon in 2:49:47 within three seconds of the same pace every mile. She lost by the race by two seconds. But, she had run a fantastic race—coming up from twentieth in the pack—and this marathon qualified Missy for Olympic Trials. She was on her way now!

By that time, running marathons had become emblazoned in her being. She knew her pace, carb intakes, insulin timing, requirements and focus. It seems hard to believe when Missy says, "I have a lazy streak in me that I have to fight every single day. I definitely think success is a great motivator though. Once you get a taste of achievement, you really don't want to lose again."

Missy tells the story about one cold, dark and rainy morning when she was training for Olympic Trials. "I had to go out for a training run and I stood in the kitchen staring out the window. My husband asked me what was wrong. And I asked him, how will I ever make it to Trials? He looked at me and replied, 'The answer's out there, not in here.'" And off she went for a sixteen mile morning run in the sleet and cold, realizing it is true—the answer is never in our cozy and warm comfort zone.

In 1999, Missy Foy became the first diabetic runner to qualify and run in the Olympic Marathon Trials. Thus far, it is an achievement she alone holds. But, it almost didn't happen. On that frantic nail-biting night before the Trials, word came down via a note to her hotel room that Missy would not be eligible to run Olympics Trials the next morning because she was using a drug, *Insulin*! A few weeks before Olympic Marathon Trials the International Olympic Committee had added insulin to its banned drug list because it is an anabolic hormone, and weight lifters and sprinters were suspected of using it to build muscle mass. The race committee at Olympic Trials quickly called in a local physician to do a physical exam to confirm that Missy did indeed have Type 1 diabetes. Because of a three-hour time difference with Colorado Springs, the wait for clearing seemed endless. Finally at 8 PM that night, just a matter of hours

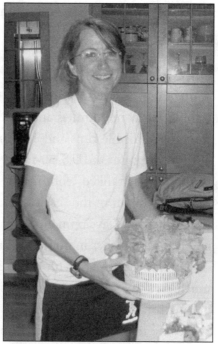

Missy's just-picked garden greens

before trials, the U.S. Olympic Committee cleared Missy for competition the next morning. Although she did not place to run in the Olympic Games, making it through trials was an astonishing achievement.

Life Must Be Paced with Balance

When not in training for an event or race, or studying, Missy enjoys the luxury of sleeping in late, enjoying the company of her great partner and husband, Bob, and their family of three stray cats. Spur-of-the-minute cookouts with friends and neighbors, and weekend chili contests, followed by fireworks on the lake, are all fun and relaxing, and help keep her life in perspective. Oh, and her all-time-favorite meal of rib-eye steak marinated in vermouth and Worcestershire, grilled over charcoal, along with a baked sweet potato with plenty of butter and sour cream, fresh green beans from her garden and a Caesar salad is a nice treat once in a while. But, truth is, she'd give up all this for a life of chocolate, very good chocolate!

Life after Qualifying for Olympic Trials

A marathon is only 26.2 miles. But, at age forty, Missy realized there were so many more miles and trails to run. That's when she began to train for fifty-mile runs and ultra marathons, and soon placed second in the country for the U.S. 50-mile National Championships! Two years prior, she was ranked tenth in the world. She has been named North Carolina Runner of the Year twice, and selected for the USA Track and Field Olympic Development Program. And on regular days? She has grabbed top finishes in numerous races across the country.

Running long—as in fifty miles long—races is a lonely life requiring much structure, accuracy and pinpoint discipline. There is no one patting you on the back to tell you what a great job you are doing when you come in sweaty and tired from a training run. You learn to pick your races, train for each specific race and connect with it. Missy is always nervous when she steps up a notch and takes on greater challenges but feels that she knows instinctually when the time is right.

In spite of some unanticipated challenges along the course, Missy has continued to successfully pursue an astounding career in distance running. Three times she has had to drop out of races due to extremes in blood sugars. On one occasion her blood sugar skyrocketed during the race. Other times, low blood sugars were the culprit. On these occasions she felt embarrassed and defeated by diabetes. As an inspiring role model, Missy talks about the ability to step out of races and not punish yourself, but sometimes it is difficult to listen to your own advice. She recalls a five mile race she lost by three-tenths of a second to her training partner. She had the race from the gun, but succumbed to the nasty fate of overconfidence. Her partner shot ahead with one hundred meters left in the race. Missy couldn't get the momentum back to win, but walked away with understanding the difference between confidence and overconfidence.

Role Model and Champion

With her vibrant personality, life experiences and winning charm, Missy generously gives of herself as a role model for other women and for children with diabetes. She counts her blessings every day. She feels privileged to have a life of running through beautiful forests. She appreciates studying subjects related to the history of medicine, which led to her receiving a Ph.D.

Being an inspiration to kids is high on Missy's priority list. She volunteers at camps where she spends quality time talking with kids on achieving their goals and taking good care of their diabetes. I remember being at a Children With Diabetes conference in Orlando a couple of years ago when Missy was speaking to a group of nine- and ten-year-olds. She told them her story of striving and working hard to become a professional athlete despite diabetes. She encouraged them to follow their dreams and focus on whatever they wanted to do. After listening rapturously to what Missy had to say, one little boy raised his hand. "How much money do you make running?" he asked. A little surprised by such a question, Missy carefully explained to the boy that at first she wasn't paid to run but through hard work she reached her goal of becoming a professional and started earning money. The boy, fist under chin, pondered this, "Nah, I don't think I want to be a runner." Missy smiled. "You might change your mind," she said, and then rustled all the kids into Sports Central gym organized by Diabetes Exercise and Sports Association. She quickly got them busy having fun running relays.

Being a role model comes with much responsibility. Missy remembers a college professor telling her that she must go on to graduate school, not because she was smart and capable but because she was a woman and had the responsibility to those who would follow in her footsteps. The professor told Missy he had three daughters who needed academic role models. He didn't want them to think the males of the species own rights to follow academic paths. The sense of confidence and pursuing dreams came to roost for Missy when she was trying to qualify for Olympic Trials. She was cautioned that a diabetic runner simply couldn't do it. If it could be done, it would have already happened. This was the moment Missy knew she *had to do it and could not fail.*

Gazing into Missy's Crystal Ball

Missy received her Ph.D. in 2013. I asked Missy about her dreams for her future, and what roads she wants to travel and road races she looks ahead to achieving.

> *I am looking forward to achieving a couple more big wins in some races and then retiring from running professionally. I'm really looking forward to having a more normal life and becoming a recreational jogger. I have been working with a couple of national caliber runners for several months now who were diagnosed with diabetes a year ago. I think one of them will become the next diabetic runner to make it to Olympic Trials. I find it very rewarding to work with them, plus it will be a huge weight off my shoulders to no longer be the only one!*

We are so fortunate to have a "sister" like Missy among us. Her banner achievements as an athlete with diabetes make us all so proud. Her kind and generous spirit and influence impact the entire diabetes community. Missy speaks of diabetes as "... having a child that never grows up. You can't go anywhere or make plans without making plans for 'the child.' I sleep with one eye open as a reminder that I have to take supplies everywhere and that a backup plan is mandatory. And, I haven't found a 'babysitter' yet I can trust." But Missy is hopeful that one day, through stem cell research, an effective way is discovered that will halt the autoimmune process that destroys beta cells, and improves our sensitivity to insulin. I say, with the greatest confidence, that everyone in the Sisterhood of Diabetes has the same rays of hope.

Thank you Missy Foy for carrying the torch for all of us!

Visit Missy's terrific website: *www.missyfoy.com*   ⟆⟅

SHAAKIRA HASSELL

She's Got What It Takes

The stories in this book all have deep roots. The women I write about live life on full tilt despite diabetes. Shaakira Hassell touched my heart with her candidness and the real way she talks about herself as an athlete facing diabetes. When I cast out the net in the diabetes community, I was looking for a sincere body of women athletes interested in telling me their stories. A letter arrived from Shaakira, a young woman from Cook County, Chicago. Here is what she wrote:

My name is Shaakira Hassell and I am contacting you in regards to the call for all sisters who are living and competing with Type 1 diabetes. I have been living with Type 1 for the past 10, almost 11 years. I was diagnosed right before I turned 21 and will be 32 this year. I am the only one in my family who is Type 1, so it was quite the anomaly when I found out. I have been an athlete all my life, so the diagnosis was a harsh blow to me and I didn't know how to manage or live with it and still compete. At the time I was playing collegiate basketball and was training to go overseas to play professionally. Needless to say, due to the newness of the diagnosis, it was a constant struggle to perform at my optimal best and continue pursuing my goal to play overseas. I still managed to acquire tryouts in Australia and for my national team in the Virgin Islands, but I still didn't feel like I was performing at my

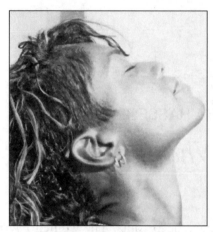

Shaakira Hassell

best even though I persevered through it (that would be the competitor in me).

Once I retired from basketball, I surprisingly picked up a pair of cleats and started playing women's professional football for the Chicago Force which is a part of the IWFL. After playing with them for a year, I moved to Georgia to pursue my Collegiate Strength and Conditioning Coaching profession with Georgia Southern University. I then moved on to Valdosta State University to continue my Master's studies. While there, I decided to play football again for the Atlanta Ravens (formerly known as the Atlanta Xplosion) women's professional football team, which was also part of the IWFL. That year we managed to overcome the odds and beat the Detroit Demolition in a heart-wrenching battle that led to us winning the IWFL National Championship in 2006. After the conclusion of that season, my career led me to Troy University in Troy, Alabama, where I have been an Assistant Speed, Strength and Conditioning Coach in the university's athletic program for four years.

So you see, Ms. Ambrosini, I think I would definitely qualify as someone who lives to compete and strives to perform despite this condition. Type 1 diabetes isn't who I am ... it's a part of the many things that I will overcome.

The Body Really Matters

When you are five-foot-eleven-inches tall and a competitive varsity basketball player, injuries are bound to be part of the game. Shaakira's junior year at Beloit College was one of those stress riddled times. In the fall of that year, 1998, she ruptured her right Achilles tendon during practice at the beginning of the season and needed serious reconstructive surgery. This injury was also a big knockout punch mentally for Shaakira since she had trained hard the previous summer with the men's basketball coach. She was in perfect shape to start a winning season.

The orthopedic surgeon told her that she would never play basketball again, but her heart told her differently. She made it clear to the doctor that *his job* was to fix the injury and, with God's help, *she* would take care of the rest.

During the period of recovery Shaakira did some research and learned that Australia was one of the top countries emerging in the field of exercise science. It also had some of the top women's pro-basketball teams. *Hmm-mm.* The wheels were spinning in Shaakira's mind. She was at this time one of the "most wanted" at the college registrar's office for not having yet declared a major. To stomp out the fires in the registrar's office, declare a major course of study and get to try out for pro-basketball overseas, she came up with the perfect solution. She created an interdisciplinary sports-science major, including a study abroad program in Australia. After much deliberation, the academic committee at Beloit gave their stamp of approval. Shaakira continued rehab for the Achilles injury throughout the spring semester and began intensive training to regain strength and condition herself for basketball again.

When she went home for the summer, she began to feel tired and fatigued all the time. She also experienced extreme thirst. She attributed it to the intensity of her power workouts. She applied for a summer job that required a physical exam. A urine analysis showed an unusually high level of ketones, a possible indicator of diabetes. This news called for major rebellion. Shaakira left the exam and bought a super-sized bag of *Sugar Babies* candy, which she proceeded to munch her way through as she drove home that afternoon.

Over the next few days the thirst became unbearable and her clothes seemed to hang off her. How could all these changes occur in such a

About Ketones

Ketones are acids that build up in the blood and spill into the urine when there is not adequate insulin on board. The body begins to burn fat instead of glucose. High ketone levels can poison the body and possibly lead to diabetic ketoacidosis (DKA), a dangerous, life threatening complication. A simple urine test using a strip similar to a glucose testing strip can detect ketones. If blood sugar levels are repeatedly over 250, it is a good idea to check for ketones. If numbers remain high for both blood sugar and ketones, it is recommended to call your doctor for further instruction.

short period of time? Worried, she went to see her primary physician who took another urine sample and blood tests which showed a 540 blood sugar. The doctor was puzzled about what kind of diagnosis to give. According to the doctor, Shaakira was too old to be Type 1 and didn't have typical Type 2 characteristics. The doctor recommended experimenting with both insulin and pills to discover which would work better. She administered a dose of insulin and gave Shaakira a prescription for meds. About an hour after she left the doctor's office, Shaakira experienced her first hypoglycemic reaction as she waited in line at the pharmacy for her prescription. In that moment of shakiness and disorientation, she knew her world would never be the same again.

Here Comes Basketball

But Shaakira was an athlete! She didn't want to become a diabetic who plays sports. For her, sports were not a hobby but a lifestyle, and she would have to figure out how to merge her competitive nature as a basketball player with the overwhelming diagnosis of diabetes.

Her introduction to basketball came at age eight when she played in an all-boys league in the inner city on Chicago's West Side. She wasn't crazy about it then, with all the running back and forth on the court, and she also resented being the only girl in the league where her father was one of the coaches.

In sophomore year at Lane Technical College Prep in Chicago, where all of her best girl friends were on the basketball team, she discovered her love for the sport. Geannetta Jackson, Shari Hayden, Sandra Urqiuiaga, Cheyenne Whitaker and the late LaShaun McKinley became the sisters Shaakira never had growing up an only child. Shaakira joined the team and basketball soon became her game. On the basketball court she discovered her unrelenting spirit and passion to persevere and overcome any odds, and she worked hard at being the best team player she could.

Not Out of the Water Yet

Shaakira was a natural athlete from the get-go. Her parents instilled the importance of physical participation and sports in their daughter at an early age. Swimming began at age five, and she played Little League baseball, studied Tae Kwon Do, ballet and gymnastics. When Shaakira was ten, her father, a teacher and administrator in the Chicago public school system for over twenty years, decided that it would be a good skill and discipline for his daughter to continue swimming until she graduated from high school. He signed her onto the YMCA swim team. The fact that Shaakira wasn't crazy about swimming held no weight. She stuck with it and became an accomplished swimmer, winning several all-city high school championships. Finally, after a successful State Championship swim meet in her senior year, she was offered scholarships to swim at several colleges. She had fulfilled her obligation to her father to stay with swimming through high school and decided to end it there because she never had the passion for swimming that she had for basketball. Instead, she accepted an academic scholarship to one of the few colleges that recruited her for basketball, Beloit College in Wisconsin. There she also had the option to compete on the swim team ... if she so desired.

Dreams Unfulfilled

Despite Shaakira's skill and talent for basketball and her fierce determination, injuries became setbacks that caused problems with her ability to play. She acquired a tryout with the Melbourne Tigers in Melbourne, Australia, during the year she spent there for her studies, then was drafted for the U.S. Virgin Islands National Basketball summer tournament in 2001. A day before reporting to the U.S. Virgin Islands, she decided to play one more pick-up game in Chicago. In a daring move during the game, she jumped to grab a rebound and landed on somebody's foot. Two days later, with a sprained ankle, she was barely able to hobble. Placed on injured reserve for the tournament, it was a hard blow for Shaakira to take after she had worked so hard to get to this point.

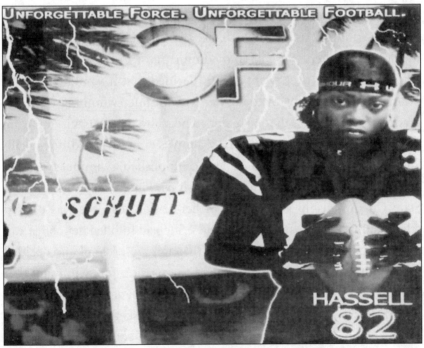

Chicago Force *Women's Professional 2004 Rookie Card*

Basketball was simply not meeting her expectations. The love turned to bitterness as she thought about the combination of her injuries and her frustrations from the difficulties of managing diabetes. Shaakira hung up her basketball shoes, ending her hopes of a longtime professional basketball career.

A New Dream Fulfilled

What did she *do* after hanging up the basketball shoes? Well, remember now that Shaakira is an athlete whose *lifestyle* is sports. So … she picked up a pair of cleats and joined the Chicago Force Women's professional tackle football team to play defensive end. To her own surprise, she fell in love with the competitive team sport of football and it soon consumed her heart and thoughts.

She continued her football career with the Atlantic Ravens (formerly the Atlanta Xplosion) during the summer season of 2006, playing defensive end and defensive tackle. That year they won the IWFL national title against the Detroit Demolition.

On the Battlefield

Diabetes has taken its toll on Shaakira for a long time. She was told by physicians that she should change her lifestyle. She was given standard issue treatments for diet and insulin that simply didn't work for her, and doctors have asked her, "Well, what do *you* think you should do?" All these factors resulted in frustration and depression. Diabetes for her has often seemed like an open wound that simply will not heal. Even after eleven years of living with diabetes, she still struggles to find the formula that works best for her. Part of this is due to having moved around from school to school and state to state. Part of it is because she has only found one doctor who really understands her level of exercise and how to manage diabetes at that extreme level.

Turning Point

When Shaakira was in Chicago, she heard about the Diabetes Exercise and Sports Association, and attended a conference at the University of Chicago in 2004. There she met Dr. Matt Corcoran, who listened to her and understood the complications of managing blood sugars with sports. She thanked God for this gift.

Shaakira realized that denying and rebelling against diabetes would get her in more trouble, so she began to come to terms with trying to manage and control it. Dr. Corcoran worked with her and gave her the confidence to pursue limitless possibilities in sports and at the same time manage her diabetes. He even supported her by attending her football games when she played pro for the Chicago Force.

Seeking a broader education, Shaakira moved to Georgia to work in the field of sports science and attain a Master's degree in Health and Physical Education from Valdosta University in 2007. She then took a position at Troy University in Troy, Alabama, as assistant coach for Speed, Strength and Conditioning. She is the coach who works behind the scenes year round to train and prepare college athletes to compete in their sports. By 2010, Shaakira had earned her second Honors Master's degree in Sports Administration at Troy, where she still works today.

Finding the Path

Although there has been much physical and emotional turbulence in Shaakira's life, she is now finding her path. With a role model like Annie Armstrong for a mother, Shaakira learned how to set goals and pursue dreams. Annie Armstrong, the strong African-American woman who served as a career soldier in the Army National Guard, and did a tour in Kuwait during Operation Enduring Freedom, wouldn't have it any other way. She completed her Master's degree in 2000 and now works for the Purple Heart of Veterans Affairs in Chicago. Shaakira learned from both her parents to prepare for success by making a plan for it and working at it with focus and determination, while using discipline to keep track of these goals.

In Shaakira's Words

Everyone has their own cross to bear; diabetes happens to be mine. I used to ask God … why me? Lord why me? until I heard His response: "Why not you? Who else better than you?" I have learned that although He has given me this cross to bear. He wouldn't give me any more than I can handle. I've learned that though I walk with this cross, He has not left, nor ever will leave my side because it is by His grace and mercy alone that I am here. He has saved me so many times that I can never deny that He does exist or that He does love and keep me in His bosom.

Despite several bouts with DKA in 2010 [Diabetic Ketoacidosis: extremely high blood sugars for a prolonged period of time, which can lead to unconsciousness, even death], Shaakira has pulled through. She recently reconnected with Dr. Corcoran to fine tune her insulin regimen and smooth out her managing skills. A renewed faith and confidence in managing diabetes and living as a power athlete is winning out. And guess what? Shaakira has returned to training as a swimmer, coming full circle back to the sport that started it all. She is working hard and hoping to compete at the U.S. Master's level. My guess is this time she'll be there one hundred percent!

The more I got to know about Shaakira, the more I felt her inspiration. I also sensed the complicated reality of living as a professional athlete dealing with the many nuances of finding the right balance between diabetes and sports. She is the role model who continues to pray, continues to fight and continues to stay strong in the battle. She told me something poignant, but rarely verbalized, that all of us living with diabetes can understand:

Not everyone understands the daily struggles we go through and how hard it is sometimes to still function in our everyday lives without wearing the face of illness even during high or low bgs. Sometimes you have to smile even though you truly feel like crying from frustration just long enough to get to a room or space by yourself to let the screams and tears out.

Part of living with diabetes is celebrating the good days and accepting the not-so-good days. But, as part of the Sisterhood of Diabetes, we get through both. We train and push the limits and win, just like our strong and persistent sister Shaakira Hassell continues to do. Thank you, Shaakira, for your inspiration. ᙠᘒ

CARLY LUDWIG

Aiming for a Hole in One with Diabetes

By age twenty-three, Carly Ludwig was a professional golfer. Her life was sparkling with a career of competition and a full agenda of good friends to have fun with when she wasn't on the golf course. Living in San Diego, Carly drifted off to sleep at night listening to the tides of the Pacific ebb and flow beyond the balcony of her bedroom. All her ducks were in a row. Life was good.

At twenty-four, Carly was a professional golfer with Type 1 diabetes. The shock of being diagnosed with diabetes at such a prime and vibrant age can cause a rapid shift in gears. Life is still good for this young native of Brownsburg, Indiana, but diabetes has changed many aspects of it.

Carly's interest in golf started when she was a twelve-year-old eighth grader. Her mom was a passionate golfer and would allow Carly to get behind the wheel and drive her golf cart. This was a major thrill, even though Carly realized she was in charge of a motorized cart and could potentially kill herself. During that time she also got to hit a ball once in a while. Carly was a natural athlete who instinctively picked up on games and sports and was always good at them. She loved competition, whether it was a team sport or she was simply competing with herself. But hitting a golf ball was another story. At age twelve she was a lousy golfer, and this really rattled her innate sense of athletics. Although she picked up on how to play the game immediately, delivering on it was another story. To Carly's sense of athletic competitiveness, this was not an acceptable way to play a sport. Golf and Carly established a love/hate relationship "right off the bat," or should I say "off the 9-iron." Still, for several months she continued to play with her mom, who convinced her to try out for the junior high school golf team, which she did. But, by the end of eighth grade, two seventh graders beat her out in scoring average. Now she was really irked. It was time for a call to arms.

Carly dove into training with all the determination and strength she had. By the end of the summer she became the only high school freshman to play varsity golf, and the first in her class to be awarded a varsity letter. At last she could live with herself again.

In the Swing of Things

Carly went on to be a successful high school player. After graduation, she played recreationally and coached for two years. While she really loved the coaching part, her longing to compete was gnawing away inside.

Off to the University of Indiana for college, she had a leg injury due to a fall that kept her in a leg cast for several weeks and necessitated her riding in a bus around campus. As a result, she began to think about moving to a warmer climate where she would be able to play golf year round. Cal State San Marcos University in San Diego proved the perfect venue. On a visit there during spring break she tried out for the team, was accepted, and soon transferred to San Diego. Here she successfully played college golf for three years.

In her senior year, Carly was an NAIA (National Association of Intercollegiate Athletics) All-American first team selection. She was on the podium in the NAIA National Championships Team in 2008, and won individual medalist in the NAIA Regional Competition that same year. In 2008, she was also awarded Player of the Year.

After graduation from college with a BS in Kinesiology and Applied Exercise Science, Carly realized that golf was meant to be the central

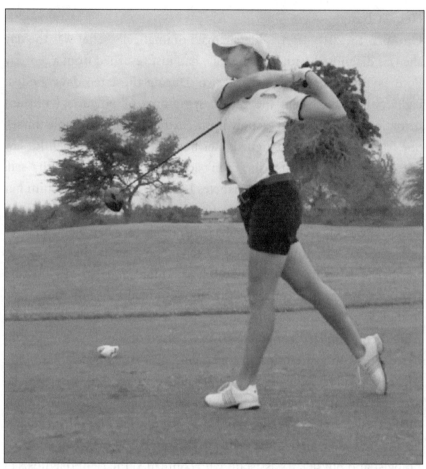

Carly Ludwig

point of her career and life. A powerful motivating force inside her drove her to compete in tournaments. And it wasn't all about winning. Carly is propelled by the exhilarating, passionate, frustrating, exciting, heart wrenching and fun times that this sport offers. Playing golf, she's in her niche. Part of that niche includes being a player at the Golden State Golf Tournament for Duramed Futures, and working as a pro player at The Santaluz Club in San Diego and as a golf sales associate at Dick's Sporting Goods. But it also means being a physical therapy aide at Core Orthopedic Center.

Game Change

On April 16, 2010, Carly's life changed dramatically. That was the day she was diagnosed with diabetes. She had just returned from a ten-day Futures Tour Tournament in Mexico. During those ten days she lost eight pounds. She had the classic symptoms of polyuria (constant urination) accompanied by polydipsia (extreme, unquenchable thirst). She felt exhausted and fatigued. Her boss was surprised when he saw her. He commented that she didn't look like her usual healthy self. He happened to have Type 1 diabetes himself. When she told him her symptoms, he whipped out his glucose meter and tested her blood sugar. The result was out of range—meaning that her blood glucose level was too high for the meter to read. She quickly found her way through a labyrinth of Urgent Care corridors and various obscure floors of the local hospital looking for some help. At last she landed in the ER, where she was diagnosed with Type 2 diabetes. The medical team there stabilized her glucose over a period of four hours, then sent her home with a prescription for Type 2 oral meds and a 300 blood sugar. A 300 blood-glucose reading is a high number, and to be given an assumed diagnosis of Type 2 diabetes without follow-up tests is not safe medical advice. (*Carly is still trying to figure out what that was all about.*) Fortunately later, after some dedicated research, she found an endocrinologist and physician's assistant who confirmed the right diagnosis of Type 1 diabetes and set her up with diabetes education, great support and insulin pump therapy.

In a flash, between the moment before and the moment after a diagnosis of diabetes, one's life changes irrevocably. Diabetes involves a big adjustment and takes time to get used to; it takes time to learn how to live with it in a positive way, particularly when it is dropped into your lap at age twenty-four. Overnight, Carly's carefree lifestyle twisted like a tornado into carb counting, insulin shots and glucose meters. She explains how it felt:

There is always some part of me that needs to be in control of my diabetes. It's hard for me to just "let go" since being diagnosed. I can't seem to relax and not worry or wonder about something related to my disease. How many carbohydrates are in this? How much insulin do I have on board? Am I going to exercise? Do I have enough sugar in case I need it? If I go low while out with my friends, will they know not to give me insulin but juice instead? Do they understand the difference between high blood sugars and low blood sugars? If I give myself insulin before bed, am I going to wake up in a low? When was the last time I ate?

Support and Elevator Music

Carly is the only one on either side of her family to have diabetes. And, even though the family is scattered about all over the country, they remain a tightly knit group who support and care for each other. Diabetes has been a learning experience for all of them.

Although Carly lives alone, there are open lines of communication between her and her family. Still it is difficult to try to explain what it is like to have this new omnipresent entity in her life that she must take care of, answer to and be aware of. As Carly says, "I sure as hell didn't grow up counting carbs and injecting insulin, and I'm glad my family didn't have to go through that phase."

Having diabetes is a learning experience. As an athlete, Carly is now more meticulous about paying attention to regulating her insulin pump, checking her blood sugar before, during, and after playing golf or exercising, and getting the right amount of carbs with some protein for energy. She carries a low-calorie sports drink on the golf course to ward off a potential drop in blood glucose. All in all she takes more precautions and is more diligent about her health.

When I asked Carly what her attitude is about diabetes, this is what she said:

This is a tough question. Maybe I don't know what I feel about having diabetes. I know a life, twenty-four years, that didn't include being a Type 1 diabetic. It didn't include a permanent prescription, insulin pump, test strips, slow acting, fast acting, gluco-tabs, highs, lows, and every other thing I am more educated about now than I ever cared to be. I have a reference point of a life I used to have. I am constantly going back and forth trying to figure out causes, reasons and inconveniences. Sometimes it exhausts me. Then I realize that Type 1 isn't the problem, it's my own perception of the disease. I am alive, I am healthy, I have a future and I can manage diabetes just fine. Every day I get the opportunity to have a better attitude about my diabetes.

So, as life goes on for this talented young professional athlete, Carly enjoys family, friends, outdoor sports, playing cards, laughing at corny jokes, playing professional golf, volunteering her services as a speaker on behalf of diabetes and exercise, plotting her future of playing golf at the highest level of her potential with her diabetes in control, and perhaps one day becoming a college coach or biomechanics professor. As an athlete, Carly's philosophy is that work is never done. "Be better, not perfect," she says. "Every day you can be better at something: a better player, better teammate, better student, better coach, and better role model. Those who succeed do so because they want to be better."

Another page from Carly's "book" of philosophy contains her caption on living with diabetes: "Diabetes is like the elevator music of my life ... always in the background and never really that great."

Carly Ludwig, you are surrounded by a sisterhood of women who are the Sisterhood of Diabetes. Our arms are open to you as we are all, along with you, role models who redefine diabetes management and try to jazz up the elevator music. ✣

CHAPTER 3

Playing For the Sport of It

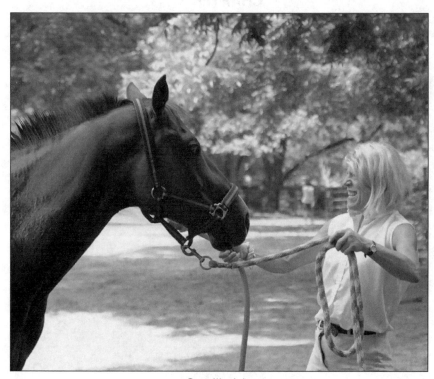

Camille Izlar

CAMILLE IZLAR

Activist, Educator, Equestrienne

Camille was told by the doctor in the hospital, "Camille, you are too sweet." This was a unique way of presenting a diagnosis of Type 1 diabetes.

The North Carolina hospital was Camille's home for two and a half weeks as she learned how to live with diabetes. There were multiple steps: administer insulin to an orange, and then carefully use an eye dropper to conduct a chemistry experiment. She placed two drops of urine into a glass test tube, followed by ten drops of water. Lastly, a pill was dropped into the mix and she watched the solution bubble up to a variety of colorful shades—from blue to orange, measuring how much sugar was spilling into her urine. When Camille was released from the hospital, she went home with ample information and confidence that she could take care of herself and lead a normal life. She was eight years old.

Camille noticed that a few things around the house had changed while she was away. Those sugar and cinnamon pop-tarts she loved had disappeared from the kitchen cabinet. It was eggs and toast for breakfast now. Oh, and at school, during cookie breaks, Camille had graham crackers for her treat; and a few times a day she'd slip into the Girls Room with her little chemistry kit to test her urine.

Her parents encouraged her to exercise and be active. She rode her bicycle up and down the street and around the corner every day after school, waiting for the day when she would be able to leave the sidewalk and venture out on the street. When that day came, she not only rode her bike in the street but she started riding horses as well. She had turned ten.

When she was thirteen, Camille's parents surprised her by buying her a horse to call her own. "Tom Terrific" was the most beautiful bay large pony in the world with his black mane and tail and white blaze. Even though he was a "mutt" (unknown breeding), he made Camille the happiest kid in town. She loved her horse and loved caring for him. For a child with a chronic disease, Tom Terrific was the perfect gift.

Forty-two years ago, at the time of Camille's diagnosis, there wasn't much in the area of education and even less information available for parents of children with diabetes. Camille's parents were both in the medical field, her father a cardiologist and her mom a registered nurse. Even though research on exercise was pale back then, they felt instinctively that activity was an important component of living a healthy life with diabetes. Hence, they nurtured and helped facilitate exercise and sports as an everyday part of Camille's young life.

At fourteen, Camille began to compete in the sport of Eventing. Eventing consists of dressage (ballet on horseback), cross country jumping (jumping about twelve to sixteen obstacles, which could consist of anything from a log to a picnic table to water, over a two-to-three mile course), and stadium jumping (jumping fences in a standard ring). Horseback riding had many positive effects on her life. Besides the rigors of being in shape physically for competition, there was the joy and responsibility of nurturing another creature—a great motivational tool for Camille.

Throughout her high school years she competed and worked at the barn where Tom lived, to help pay for the upkeep of her horse. Although Tom Terrific was her passion, Camille also managed to run track and was a member of the cheerleading squad. Once she entered the University of Virginia, however, she realized she had to line up her priorities. Unfortunately, due to distance and money, she had to let go of her beloved pony and riding.

Going off to college generally means leaving the nest and flying tenuously towards independence, and this can have many effects on a young student. For children who have lived with diabetes since they were youngsters, this sense of freedom can tumble into a false sense of "freedom" from diabetes. Camille went through a period of denial, not testing blood sugars, drinking and eating to excess, in other words, following the crowd. She chose to hide her diabetes because of the element of shame associated with a chronic condition such as diabetes. This disease can make you feel imperfect in the eyes of fellow students who were not educated on the subject. Truth is, with a little more planning, those of us with diabetes can conquer the same mountain tops as everyone else. In Camille's case, she learned to use diabetes as a motivation to move forward with a positive attitude.

Commitment to the Diabetes Community

The diabetes community became a focal point for Camille. Although medical school had been the original goal, her work at a summer diabetes camp—where she taught children how to manage their diabetes—pointed her toward a career in diabetes education. After receiving a degree in psychology at the University of Virginia, Camille went on to a Master's program in nutrition at the University of North Carolina, Greensboro. Since then she has amassed an impressive list of degrees and certifications beyond college: MS, RD, LDN (licensed dietitian/nutritionist), CDE and BC-ADM (Board certified in Advanced Diabetes Management). Camille has dedicated her life and career to helping others with diabetes.

She told me:

I eat, sleep and drink diabetes. Diabetes is part of who I am. When I was younger I didn't like having diabetes and didn't want people to know about it until I proved myself, in other words showed them that I could do anything they did. These days I think people realize that those of us who live with diabetes can do anything we set our dreams on. What they don't know is all it takes to make those dreams happen. But, yes we can do anything.

Camille lived in Winston-Salem, North Carolina, and worked as a diabetes educator at Bowman Gray Medical Center, Wake Forest University. Then, in 1990, five years after grad school, she bought another horse and named it Jackson (for Jackson, Wyoming, where she honeymooned). Her passion for animals, riding and competition were back, and so she trained Jackson and started competing again ... but not for long. Circumstances forced Camille to give up Jackson, and shortly afterward she moved back to where she grew up and again took a job working full time as a diabetes educator and clinical instructor at the University of North Carolina School of Medicine.

Camille did not have a horse for about two years. But after a trip out west to Nevada, while riding across the mountain ranges outside of Reno, she decided she needed another horse in her life. As it turned out, when she returned home, a friend found her a baby horse that needed a home, and so began a new horse adventure in 2003 with "Nevada Joy," an eighteen-month-old quarter horse mare. Since then Camille has been competing with Nevada in the sport of Eventing.

Working full time and preparing for competition by riding everyday can be brutal at times, but when you are as passionate about something as Camille is about riding, you do whatever it takes. In a way, the daily discipline of checking blood sugars, counting carbs, maintaining a healthy and balanced diet, staying involved with exercise and sports and always having backup plans are helpful in many avenues of life. As Camille says, "Use diabetes as a prod, not as a crutch."

Along with her passion for the equestrian arts, Camille has run two marathons and two half-marathons, and in the process raised over $20,000 for diabetes research. In 2001, during the Rome Marathon (her first), she ran the first thirteen miles over ancient cobblestone streets in the center of old Rome with a Type 1 teammate who needed to make frequent stops throughout the 26.2 mile course. Seven hours later, the pair joyfully crossed the finish line and Camille had blisters on just about every toe. Chalk one up for her first marathon! Her second 26.2 run came in 2002 in Dublin, Ireland. Her two half-marathons were in Bermuda and Kona, Hawaii. All of these races were part of Team Diabetes events, which means that many of the runners involved also had diabetes. Needless to say, Camille was in

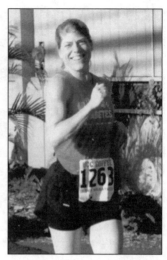

Camille runs, too

good company. Running continues to be part of her daily life, and when there is a worthy cause to help raise funds for diabetes research, she is compelled to train for it and give it her very best. After all, the research must go on in hopes that one day a cure will be found.

Challenges to Life with Diabetes

Camille has seen many changes and much progress in diabetes management in the forty-two years she has lived with Type 1 diabetes. Although her life with diabetes has been quite extraordinary and filled with devotion and responsibility to help others, there has been some sadness also. Life is rarely walked on a straight line or run at the perfect pace. Something that brings Camille great sorrow is that she never had children. When she was married and got pregnant, she was told by the so called experts of the day that it was neither safe nor wise, and that the risk was too high for Type 1 diabetics to bear children. There were other complications, like her diabetic retinopathy which had been treated with laser and followed with vitrectomy surgery in both eyes. And so, she did not continue with the pregnancy. This type of advice was common years ago.

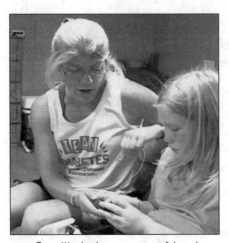

Camille helps a young friend

Today we know better. Thanks to endocrinologists such as Lois Jovanovic (also a Type 1) who studied fifty-two Type 1 subjects through pregnancy. Her published research, in 1981, in the *Journal of American Medicine*, showed that with constant monitoring and tight control, women with Type 1 diabetes could give birth to healthy babies. Dr. Jovanovic has since developed a precise protocol that has helped women worldwide maintain excellent blood glucose levels during pregnancy. Her work has helped change the once frightening uncertainty of diabetes and pregnancy. Today, useful technology such as insulin pumps and continuous glucose monitors are terrific aids that result in healthy babies. In the "stone age" of diabetes care, Camille along with other women, this writer included, were unfortunate victims of the times.

Camille Izlar, activist, educator and equestrian leads a full and rich, dedicated and responsible life. To have diabetes, to live with it as part of who you are and then jump that hurdle, that fence, and dedicate yourself to teach and counsel others in how to manage their diabetes, takes a strong, bright light that glows from within this enlightened diabetes educator. Camille believes that part of God's plan for her is to use her diabetes to help others with diabetes. She teaches by example that you can do anything … just be sure you are prepared … because sometimes there are bumps in the road. Camille cautions, "Don't turn the bumps into mountains."

Thank you, Camille, for sharing your light, your life and your story with us. Your friends and fellow travelers in the Sisterhood of Diabetes salute you!   ✎✎

EMILY IANNELLO TIBERIO

The Ice Hockey Engineer

There are a few things you know about when you come from Buffalo, New York: snow, chicken wings, how to lose consecutive Super bowl games, and the Buffalo Sabres ice hockey team. Emily Iannello Tiberio hadn't missed a Sabres game since she was a kid, whether she went to see them play, watched them on TV or listened to the games on the radio. She was from Buffalo and she was a hockey fan.

Street hockey was big in my neighborhood in Buffalo. I was the only girl who played and I was one of the toughest players. I loved hockey from the first time I picked up a stick that I borrowed from a boy down the street. My family moved to West Seneca, a Buffalo suburb, and the town started its first girls' ice hockey club. I begged and begged my parents to let me play. My mom said I'd get all my teeth knocked out. I didn't join the club. Instead I became a soccer goalie, ran mid-distance track and played lacrosse—sports that kept me moving for every season from middle school through high school.

But Emily loved ice hockey, and really wanted to skate.

As time went on, Emily continued to play sports in a powerful and energetic way. She received a BS in Electrical Engineering Technology from Rochester Institute of Technology, where she played one year of intercollegiate soccer and four years of lacrosse. The day after graduation, the first thing she did was run downtown to a used sporting goods store to buy her first set of hockey equipment.

Emily went on to work at RE Ginna Nuclear Power Plant in Ontario, New York, where she began her career as an instruments and controls electrical systems engineer. She continued to work in that position for three years. During that time she discovered that the wife of one of her fellow engineers belonged to a Hockey Moms Club, where the moms of a bunch of the hockey players were learning how to skate and play the game just like their kids did. They accepted Emily as an honorary mom and invited her to play with the club. The

A Few Words About Women and Hockey

Since the 1990s, the face and gender of ice hockey has become more noticeable with a substantial interest from girls and women. There are co-ed teams, female leagues and intercollegiate tournaments. Women's hockey is now an official Olympic sport. Seems like this is something new, doesn't it? Actually it was in the 1890s when female hockey teams began playing. There are two records of the first female hockey games; one is from the Canadian Hockey Association, which claims the first game was played in Barrie, Ontario, in 1892. The official NHL records show the first game as the 1889 game when the Government House team defeated the Rideau Ladies in Ottawa. We may never know which really came first.

Women's hockey enjoyed its heyday in the 1920 and '30s when the Preston Ontario Rivolettes dominated the game as national champions in Canada throughout that period. After that, hockey returned to being a predominantly male sport. In fact, in 1956, a nine-year-old girl, Abbie Hoffman, who had played most of the season on an all-boys minor team, challenged the "all-boys" policy in court. She had disguised herself by wearing short hair, and she dressed at home for games; all in all, Abbie was a terrific part of the team. However, the Ontario Supreme Court ruled against her participation in this "all-boys" sport.

It was a long slow battle, but women finally won the war. Women's intercollegiate hockey became accepted, and in 1993 the NCAA recognized women's hockey as a legitimate sport. In 1998, women's hockey debuted in the Japan Olympics. In 2002, another breakthrough occurred when the Mission Bettys of California became the first all-girls team to enter one of the world's largest youth competitions, the Quebec International Pee Wee Tournament. In 2003, Hayley Wickerheiser became the first woman to score a point on a men's professional hockey team.

Although Canada and the U.S. remain dominant in the field, in a landmark playoff game in the 2006 Olympics, Sweden took the silver medal. Goaltender Kim Martin was cheered as the new face of women's hockey. Girls and women's hockey is rapidly reclaiming its place as a popular international sport.

dream of playing hockey had at last come true.

Emily on Ice

Perhaps because she knew the game so well and had been a lifelong hockey fan, Emily took to the ice immediately and with great gusto. She learned to play at last … just as she had always dreamed of doing. While she continued to play hockey with the Hockey Moms for a while, Emily soon realized that she needed a faster and tougher game than what they played, despite the fact that they had changed their name to "Slapshot Sisters." After a little investigation, she signed up with an intermediate-level men's hockey league named "The Misfits." Still practicing with the Slapshot Sisters, her game with the men's league kept improving, and soon she also started up a hockey team at work, the "Ginna Nukes," who played in a local league and against other nuclear power plants. She is still the only female among the three teams at work, but is hoping that will change.

Emily is one of the hardest working players in the league today. During her second season with the Misfits, Emily met Dan Tiberio, another avid hockey player and fan. Emily and Dan married in November 2010 in Niagara Falls, New York, where, at the wedding, they skated their first dance together on a synthetic ice rink!

Life with Diabetes

On March 4, 2008, at age twenty-four, Emily entered her doctor's office with a laundry list of symptoms:

- 10 lbs. underweight
- drinking approximately five gallons of water daily
- dehydrated
- exhausted and fatigued

The doctor gave her a prescription for blood work, and told her he would call her with the results. But Emily was too stubborn to wait for an answer. She knew her body and knew something wasn't right. The doctor gave her the option that, "if she felt that strongly about it," he could call for an ambulance to take her to the ER immediately.

An ambulance ride was not on Emily's life bucket list, so instead she went home and packed an overnight bag and drove herself to the ER in the middle of the afternoon. After waiting several hours, she described her symptoms to the nurse who did a blood glucose reading. The meter beeped abruptly and read CRITICAL HIGH. The nurse turned to Emily and in a matter of fact tone of voice stated, "Honey you're diabetic!" Emily let her know immediately that this was *totally impossible*. There was no diabetes in her family; she was a healthy athlete; and she always took good care of herself.

Emily sat alone on a chair for hours in the hallway of the ER waiting for a bed. If it was true she had diabetes, she didn't want it. She didn't want to be sick. It made no sense at all.

As she waited, she fought off tears with every bit of energy she could muster. Finally, she was plugged into an IV to treat her dehydration. A couple of hours later, when a bed became available, blood drawings began, along with a barrage of other tests.

People from work started calling to find out where she was and what was going on. Emily remembers clearly:

I had been in the ER the entire day and still hadn't called my parents. I couldn't just call and say, "Hey, yeah I'm in the ER and I'm not sure what's wrong with me. They're running tests." So I waited until the test results came in that night before calling my mother to tell her I had been diagnosed with Type 1 diabetes— which she didn't believe. I didn't let her and my dad drive to see me that night. It was already late and I felt really exhausted. They came the next day as I was in the process of getting released. The nurse was trying to show me how to give myself a shot with a Quick Pen, and teaching me how to use a meter to test my blood sugar. My new endocrinologist told me that the only reason he was releasing me from the hospital so soon—most newly diagnosed patients stayed one week—was because I was the first patient who asked for books and printouts and graph paper to start learning how to take care of myself and how to track my progress.

Emily's parents stayed with her for the first few days trying to understand their daughter's new diagnosis and coping with it themselves. It took her forty-five minutes to administer her first insulin shot by herself; it was hard to see the needle through her tears. As the first traumatic week wound down, the engineer in her took over. Food charts and diagrams became part of her daily routine as she turned herself

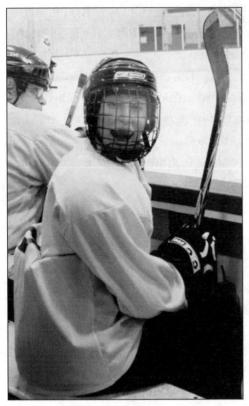
Emily, ready for the ice

into a science experiment. Emily was determined *not* to let diabetes control her busy life. *She* would be in control.

Those first few months were a real roller coaster ride of emotions and physical stress, trying to figure out what it meant to be diabetic, and what it meant to be a healthy one. She poured over books and Internet sites, and shared everything she learned with Dan, her family, friends and co-workers. As a result, Emily's support system learned about everything she did about her diabetes. They even listened patiently to the results of her blood sugar readings. They kept her motivated and positive. The Iannello family pulled out their grab-bag of characteristic humor to keep her laughing. For instance, one of Emily's little cousins was witness to a frustrating "diabetic moment" at a family reunion last summer. He turned her tears of frustration into tears of laughter when he teased … "Diabetes? It's more like CRY-abetes! Emily has CRY-abetes!"

Diabetes is still something new to Emily, but she has great hopes and big plans for the future. Gone are the days when, after being diagnosed, she would decide she could take "diabetes-free" vacation days without checking blood sugars or taking insulin. Emily says, "I think I did this because I was still coping with my diabetes and still felt like a freak show about it. I feel much better about it all now, and keep diabetes with me constantly."

Emily and Dan have started a family. She continues to work in her field but is considering stepping away from the engineering world to go back to school for a new dual career, combining motherhood and something diabetes related, so she can help people be as happy and healthy as she has become. She would also like to start up a group in the Rochester area for diabetic athletes. This group will not only organize sporting events, it will encourage those at various stages of coping with diabetes who are hesitant or just starting out with exercise and sports.

In the meantime, Emily continues with her passion for hockey, runs half-marathons, practices yoga, plays kickball with a group of co-workers, and plays even more hockey on weekends with friends. For several summers she managed to squeeze in time to coach Lacrosse to third and fourth grade girls. Then, she got the job of head coach of the junior varsity girls' lacrosse team at Webster Schroeder high school for the spring 2010 season. Teaching eighth through eleventh graders is a different challenge from teaching third and fourth graders, but she finds it rewarding and lots of fun.

Skates Off—Running Shoes On

Emily's first diabetic half-marathon in Buffalo on May 25, 2008, a little over two months after her diagnosis, was a huge milestone for her, and she finished strong with no blood sugar complications. May 2009 was even better with the aid of a continuous glucose monitoring system and a personal best race finish time of 1:51:09. At the finish line she cried with joy.

In August 2010, Emily marked her two-year anniversary of diabetes with a new challenge. She participated in twenty-four-hour relay race from Winona, Wisconsin, to Minneapolis, Minnesota, with a team made up of eleven other Type 1s from across North America. The

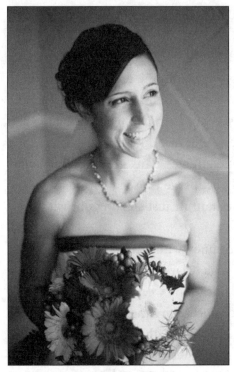

Emily Iannello Tiberio

team represents Glucomotive, *www.glucomotive.org*, a non-profit running and walking organization for people with diabetes. Emily ran a total of fifteen miles in each of three legs of the 193.2 mile relay. Currently, Emily has taken on leadership roles with both Glucomotive and Insulindependence organizations.

About accepting challenges, Emily says:

The tubes from your insulin pump are not tying you down, they are setting you free. Also, it's okay to have bad days. Everyone has bad days. You can't be perfect with your diabetes. You can try, but it won't work all the time. Accept the fact that there will be days when you do everything right and your blood sugars still don't turn out the way you expected them to. Accept the fact that every once in awhile you'll have to stop running or stop skating to take care of yourself and take care of your blood sugar. There is nothing wrong with putting yourself first. The finish line will still be there and you can go back to work, getting there after your blood sugar is under control.

Thank you, Emily Iannello Tiberio, goaltender and goal setter, for being part of the Sisterhood of Diabetes. We wish you the best! ✞

ULRIKE THURM

"Can't" Means ... "Yes, I Can"

Ulrike Thurm, a native of Westfalen, Germany, was diagnosed with Type 1 diabetes when she was twenty-one years old. That was twenty-six years ago.

She started playing sports as a young girl. In fact, by age five, Ulrike had her eyes set on becoming a professional soccer player, and she played soccer every day with the neighborhood boys. The only stumbling block in her plan was that, at that time, soccer was a boys-only sport in Germany. But Ulrike loved the game so much that she came up with an idea of how she could continue to play. She decided to disguise herself as a boy and try out for a local team.

Things were going quite well during the workout, but the fatal blow came for Ulrike after training was over, when the team was required to go into the locker room for showers. She had to admit she was Ulrike (a girl's name) and not Uli (a boy's name), and thus her soccer career was over before it even began.

But that was many years ago. Things have changed, and women's soccer is now a popular sport in Germany with both European and World Championship wins. Although Ulrike is not a professional player, since she started playing in soccer leagues at a time when many professionals were nearing retirement, today she plays defense on some highly competitive soccer teams in Berlin.

The All-Rounder

I wondered what Ulrike's life was like after she found out, at age five, that she couldn't play professional soccer. She told me that her love of sports exposed her to many different interests. She loved horseback riding and played handball as a young girl. As she grew up, it was tennis and long distance running. She became a good swimmer and scuba diver. She cycled and enjoyed in-line skating. Always good at every sport she played, Ulrike thinks of herself as an "all-rounder"—meaning she's good at everything, but not great at any one in particular.

When Ulrike, an only child, was thirty-four, her father passed away. That same year her mother had a stroke and Ulrike took care of her as best she could for many years. Her mother was a strong-willed woman and a fighter, driving around in her motorized wheelchair and able to manage her life joyfully. It was difficult for Ulrike when, in the winter of 2012, her mother passed away. But Ulrike has inherited her mother's "fighter" gene and become a force to be reckoned with in her career and on the playing field.

The Field Broadens

Ulrike went to university to study mathematics, sports and German with the intention of becoming a teacher. However, when she was diagnosed with Type 1 diabetes at age twenty-one, she shifted her course. At that time physical education teachers with Type 1 diabetes were not granted a certification to teach. So Ulrike chose to become a diabetes specialist nurse—a new beginning for her. She got the opportunity to study under a renowned German endocrinologist, Dr. Michael Berger, at University Hospital in Düsseldorf. Dr. Berger was one of the most famous researchers in the field of diabetes and exercise at the time. In 1989, he was invited to England to speak at the first International Diabetic Athletes Association (IDAA) conference, and Ulrike went with him. She was so enthralled by the concept and philosophy of having an organization for diabetic athletes that she expressed her wish to organize a chapter in Germany. Dr. Berger agreed with her and committed to help in any way he could.

    The timing was right. IDAA England planned a coast-to-coast relay run for a team of diabetic runners. The goal was to complete the run in under twenty-four hours. Ulrike was so keen on the idea that Dr. Berger offered to pay her airfare to England if she trained hard enough to make the team. She set out with her typical enthusiasm and determination and was chosen for the team. In addition, Ulrike launched IDAA Germany.

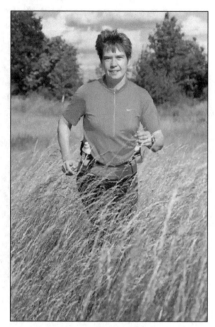

Ulrike Thurm

The following year, 1990, the World Health Organization (WHO) meeting on diabetes and exercise took place in Düsseldorf, bringing all the major experts in the field to this conference. Ulrike wanted to show this group of scientists and clinicians that when a diabetic athlete hears the word "*Can't*" it translates to "*Yes, We Can!*" To this end she organized a non-stop bicycle tour from Mainz to Düsseldorf—roughly 300K (180 miles). The plan was to begin the ride at midnight in Mainz and arrive in Düsseldorf in time to open the conference. In Ulrike's words:

> *Paula Harper, founder of IDAA, and Angelo Centeno, a blind cyclist from New York City, were with us to support the opening of the German chapter of IDAA. What a night it turned out to be with blind Angelo singing on the back of his tandem as we all cycled down the Rhine. We pulled in to open the conference the next day with great cheers and enthusiasm from the crowd. I think most of them had doubted that a non-stop bike tour of*

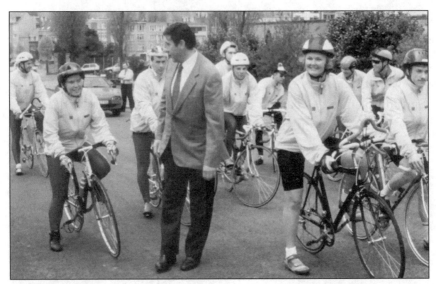

Ulrike Thurm   Paula Harper

this length would be possible for athletes with Type 1 diabetics.
We sure proved a thing or two! The scientists began to understand
the abilities within the patient with diabetes. We all celebrated the
event with champagne and a wonderful dinner. I will never forget
those twenty-four hours.

A Guiding Light

Since 1990, the German IDAA group of athletes with diabetes has
grown stronger and steadily under Ulrike's commanding guidance.
She publishes and edits a yearly magazine-length newsletter. She has
written two books, one on diabetes and exercise and one on continuous glucose monitoring and insulin pump therapy. Both books
are standards for all Type 1s in Germany today. As a member of the
German Diabetes Association, she has authored guidelines on how
to treat diabetes during exercise and sport. The publication is called
Leitlinien. Under Ulrike's direction, the German chapter also posts
many outstanding sporting activities.

In 1992, the group was invited to attend the Olympics in Barcelona. Ulrike got busy, and with support from Boehringer Mannheim, a German pharmaceutical company, she organized a bike tour from Brussels to Barcelona. The team consisted of twelve Type 1 cyclists from eleven countries. As the group cycled into Barcelona, they were welcomed by a police escort in cars and on motorcycles, and accompanied to the Olympic stadium where the Olympic organizing committee presented them with real Olympic medals. That was quite a memorable day for these athletes, and Ulrike was so proud of all of them and for the recognition.

Scuba diving was a sport that had been banned in Germany for people with insulin dependent diabetes. To change this law, Ulrike arranged a research project in Papua, New Guinea, with help from American Steve Prosterman, a Type 1 scuba diver. The research *proved* that this sport was safe for divers with insulin dependent diabetes. Back home in Germany the ban was lifted, and Ulrike initiated courses for scuba diving trainers to learn about special features to include when teaching diving courses to people with diabetes. That was in 1995. Since then, scuba diving has become a safe and popular sport for insulin-dependent diabetics.

The year before the scuba diving research, Ulrike went to Austria to study blood glucose testing at heights of 4000 meters above sea level. The research team climbed and ran in the mountains as part of their studies. Ulrike also spent one year in Australia where she cycled through the Australian desert from Perth to Alice Springs in the name of diabetes research. While there, Ulrike met Australian champion Type 1 cyclist Monique Hanley, who agreed to form an Australian IDAA chapter. It has since evolved to become the booming organization "Hypoactive," as noted in Chapter 2.

Through the years, Ulrike put into play a systemized support arena for diabetic runners in the Berlin Marathon. That began in 2002 and continued for several years. These days, she and her group follow all the big marathons throughout Germany, hosting the diabetic runners. In 2011, a marathon in Cologne had more than one hundred Type 1 and Type 2 runners participating, including Ulrike, who is always one of the athletes who run. In 2013, the group ran Berlin again. This support group is part of the official medical team, and they are always surprised at the ability of people with diabetes to run marathons so well.

One fond memory Ulrike cherishes is the time she ran the Berlin Marathon with her friend Heinz who was celebrating a successful fifty years of living with Type 1 diabetes. It was his first marathon, and Ulrike ran with him until the two of them joined hands and crossed the finish line together.

It Always Goes Back to Soccer

Since the beginning of the biennial International Diabetes and Exercise conferences in 1989, each meeting has been held in a different country. The inevitable highlight on the closing day is a fiercely competitive soccer game. The two teams are "Italy" against the "Rest of the World." Inevitably, by the end of the match, everyone in attendance has lost

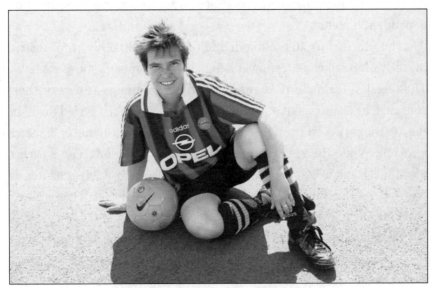

Ulrike, soccer coach and player

Global Hero for One Day

When it was suggested to Ulrike that she apply for the "Medtronic Global Heroes" award program, she couldn't imagine why, despite the fact that she is a marathoner, cyclist, soccer and tennis player, and licensed rescue diver. Medtronic is a medical device company that makes everything from implantable defibrillators to pace makers to insulin pumps. Ulrike wears a Medtronic Minimed insulin pump and CGM device (continuous Glucose Monitor).

Candidates for the award are judged by a non-partisan marathon committee not Medtronic. The purpose of the Heroes program is to celebrate the passion and accomplishments of runners who benefit from medical technology.

Once she found out that the Heroes ceremony would take place at the hilly Twin Cities Marathon from Minneapolis to St. Paul—with a four-mile mountain challenge at mile nineteen—her interest really piqued. There was also the motivating fact that no German had ever been chosen for this honor.

The good news of Ulrike's acceptance arrived in Berlin on her birthday in 2010. It was a wonderful birthday present. The 26.2 mile run would be grueling for this seasoned athlete of twelve marathons because of the altitude and mountains involved in the event. But, as Ulrike put it: "If you want to be a hero you can't let a couple hills scare you." And so with rigorous training and careful monitoring of blood sugars, she was well prepared for the run.

In Minneapolis, she met all the other Global Heroes representing every continent. The early October run allowed her a breathtakingly beautiful vista of autumn in the American Midwest, with throngs of well-wishers cheering all along the route. At the finish line, Medtronic welcomed the Heroes as their names were announced over the loudspeaker, and the enthusiastic crowds cheered for each of them.

Ulrike *felt* like a Hero that day as she proudly wore her "Global Hero" shirt, crossing the finish line in 4:40 despite running through mountains with good blood sugars and a CGM and Medtronic insulin pump.

their voices from cheering so loudly, and Italy always wins. That is, until 2008 at the University of Toronto. Team Italy, as ever, was dressed in their national colors. The Rest of the World team wore … well we won't even discuss the colors or shirts they wore. But it wasn't about uniforms or the torrential rains that fell that afternoon. It was about the passion of both teams of diabetic athletes, and the tough-as-nails little fighter who coached and played with them, that brought the Rest of the World to victory for the first time. You know who I mean? The little girl from Westfalen, Germany, who wanted to be a professional soccer player at age five—Ulrike Thurm.

Ulrike is a true inspiration to all those she meets and works with, and we are honored and so proud to have her amongst us in The Sisterhood of Diabetes. In November 2012, Ulrike came to New York to run the marathon, only to find that the race had been cancelled due to the devastation from Hurricane Sandy. This didn't stop her from running a marathon. She ran the "historic" original New York marathon route of four loops around Central Park!   ⊱♡

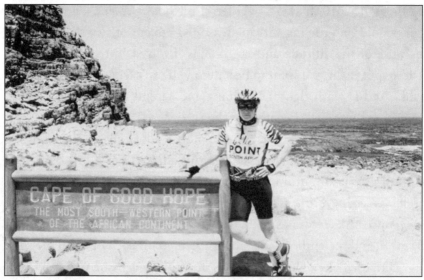

Ulrike may turn up anywhere!

NICOLE MARCELIN

From Dragon Boats to Everest Base Camp

Consider diabetes in everything you do because it's relevant, but don't ever let it hold you back. I've traveled to dozens of countries, competed in cross country running, Nordic ski racing, soccer, field hockey, ultimate Frisbee and dragon boat racing. I have flown across time zones, studied in Germany, swam in several oceans and many lakes wearing my insulin pump, eaten curries in Thailand, Nepal and India, run dozens of 10k races and a half-marathon, snowboarded at Whistler Mountain and trekked to base camp at Mt. Everest. You can, too.

This, my friends, is Nicole Marcelin.

Nicole was diagnosed with Type 1 diabetes four days prior to her fifth birthday. She spent that birthday at Children's Hospital of Eastern Ontario. She never played sports in elementary school except when required, but a program called "Canada Fitness Testing" that encouraged children to be physically active attracted her, and in eighth grade Nicole was presented with an excellence award medal in the 2400 meter run. This honor inspired her to join cross country running the following year as a high school freshman. With a great coach—Mr. Brereton—and fantastic teammates, the cross country team made it to the provincial championships that year. Although Nicole never thought of herself as being competitive or even athletic, the experience of being part of a winning team that year sealed her destiny as a committed and serious athlete.

On Becoming a Competitive Athlete

Hard work punctuated with achievement as a young teenager continued to guide Nicole's philosophy and lifestyle all the way from running 2k the first day of cross country practice to completing a half marathon. At the end of the season, another coach, Ms. Terrett, recognized Nicole's ability and encouraged her to try out for cross country skiing. This same sense of working toward goals and giving it her best as an athlete and team player cascaded into ski racing throughout all her years of high school. With Ms. Terrett pushing Nicole towards other sports, she joined the soccer and field hockey teams and enjoyed both.

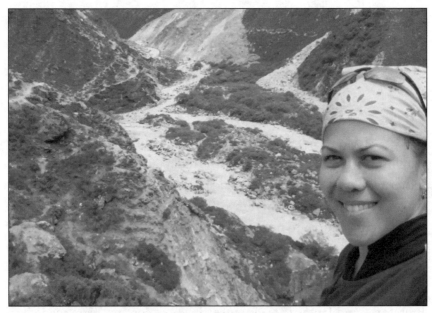

Nicole Marcelin

During university summers in Ottawa, Nicole experienced the thrill of dragon boat racing and loved it. From the start, she knew that one day she would be racing competitively rather than just for fun.

When Nicole moved to Vancouver to begin a career in the diabetes world for LifeSccan, a J&J company that makes One-Touch glucose strips and meters for home monitoring, she landed in her "spot." The company had an established dragon boat team. Nicole joined the team and found it a perfect match for her with its balance of competitiveness and camaraderie. The team went on to participate in several international competitions (which they call "festivals). They competed in Hong Kong in 2012, as well as U.S. competitions in Portland and Seattle. As of 2013, they had competed at the Kaiser Permanente San has made it to the largest Division A festivals in the U.S.

This sport continues to motivate and thrill Nicole.

DRAGON BOAT RACING

Traditionally, a "dragon boat" is a human powered water craft made of teak wood from the Pearl River delta region of Southern China. Its size and design vary. Dragon boats are one type of several varieties of long boats commonly found in Asia, Africa and the Pacific Islands. A team paddling sport, its roots trace back over 2000 years as part of ancient folk festivals and religious rituals. Modern dragon boat racing has emerged as an international sport organized by the International Dragon Boat Federation. The standard crew of a contemporary dragon boat is twenty-two teammates consisting of twenty paddlers in pairs facing toward the bow of the boat, one drummer or caller at the bow facing toward the paddlers, and one sweep (who steers) at the rear of the boat. Races are usually 500 meters in length with teams competing against other boats in several heats throughout a day or weekend of exciting races.

What About Diabetes?

With all the amazing things that Nicole does, she balances her diabetes well. Having been diagnosed at such a tender age, she has never known any other way. Because of this, she eats wholesome foods, stays attuned with all the cutting-edge diabetes technology, and works in the diabetes community; and about exercise … well, she certainly gets plenty of that. If she's not dragon boat racing, she's running with friends or lifting weights or taking boot camp sessions at the gym.

Nicole feels best when she's outdoors, and she found a golden opportunity to be "about as outdoors as you can get" as part of a team of hikers with Type 1 diabetes who trekked for ten days to the base camp of the highest spot on this planet, Mt. Everest. There she soon learned that spending time in high altitude and trekking for days is taxing for *any* person. Add managing diabetes to the mix and you are presented with some extra challenges. The body reacts strangely in altitude, increasing insulin resistance despite the intense physical effort required to do simple things like walking. Frequent blood sugar monitoring was needed to insure that basal rates and even bolus ratios increased adequately to avoid hyperglycemia.

Nicole imagined that after her exhilarating and strenuous experience of Everest, she would be on a "superhero" level of physical fitness and strength. Indeed she was super fit, but more than that. The extreme mental focus required every minute, in simply putting one foot in front of the other, taking one small step at a time, with no possibility to go back or rush forward, inspired a toughness and strength in her that has translated into better endurance running and dragon boat paddling.

The Framework of Nicole's Life

Diabetes frames Nicole's life. As she tells me:

> I never forget I have diabetes. It frames almost every thought I
> have … how I'm feeling, where my blood sugars are going, what

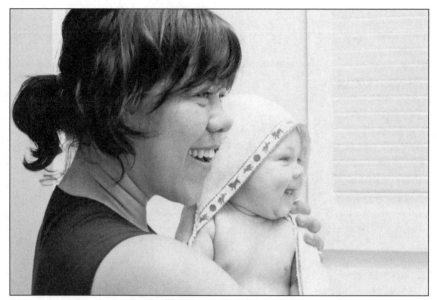

Nicole Marcelin and Leila

I'm going to eat, when I'm going to exercise and what effect stress or sickness is going to have on my blood sugars. It's always there. It is also a way to stay alert and not take any details for granted. I sometimes think that this attention to detail makes me nervous or anxious. But then I say to myself, that's how I roll.

Nicole's life is not always filled with dragon boats and treks to Mt. Everest. It is balanced with love of family, her mate Adrian, and precious baby Leila. Her wish is for them to always live happily and healthily.

Nicole said at the beginning of her story, "Consider diabetes in everything you do because it is relevant, but don't ever let it hold you back." And she hasn't. We are exhilarated by her inspiring life. Thank you, Nicole Marcelin. Perhaps one day we might just be lucky enough to run into you as we venture on the pathway of the Sisterhood of Diabetes.   ⊰⊱

CHAPTER 4

Strength and Power Inside and Out

JEN HANSON

With a Smile and a Headlock

Put on sweats…
Wrap up like a mummy in plastic wrap…
Slip into several layers of oversized plastic bags…
Climb many, many flights of stairs…
Run in place in a sauna or steam room while desperately sucking
on ice cubes…

What some people do for the thrill of participating in competitive sport! In the rough and tumble sport of wrestling, making-weight or weight-cutting to qualify for particular classifications can get really hot! Who would contrive such bizarre rituals? Who would be driven to actually do them on a regular basis?

Jen Hanson would, and did, with a smile and a headlock.

The Wrestling Game

Wrestling began for Jen in sixth grade in Sunderland, Ontario, when a team was formed at the elementary school she attended. The school offered all kinds of exciting and innovative sports, and wrestling was one of them. Jen and a few of the other girls went for it. It turned out that Jen was good, and so she continued to wrestle through high school and university years. During this time she wrapped, sweated and sucked on ice cubes to make qualifying weight for competitive matches as a member of both her high school and university varsity wrestling teams. For elementary and most of high school wrestling, cutting weight wasn't an official requirement, but since the older, "cooler" wrestlers did it, it seemed like the thing to do.

As the eldest in a family of five kids, competition came naturally. Wrestling was not Jen's first sport, however. First was ballet class, and gymnastics and soccer soon followed. The stakes grew as Jen did— hockey, rugby, wrestling and ringette, which is similar to hockey but much faster. So, what started out as ballet class evolved into Jen joining the high school wrestling team, and then being recruited and offered an academic scholarship to Brock University in St. Catharines, Ontario, where she made the varsity wrestling team. As it happened, Brock was a national training center for the sport, and many of Jen's teammates competed for the Canadian Olympic team.

Female Olympic wrestling has four stringent weight classes: 48 kg., 55 kg., 63 kg., and 72 kg. Men's has a broader scope and larger number of classifications. The class that Jen competed in was not within those qualifying

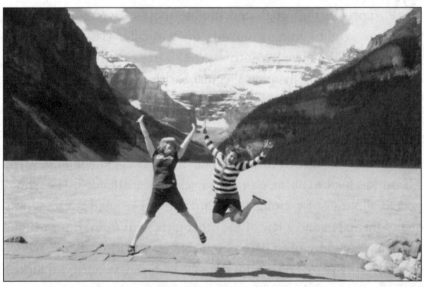

Jen Hanson (right) and friend in the Canadian Rockies

boundaries. Several of her teammates chose to drop large amounts of weight over time to make the lower qualifying weight, but this was not something Jen had a burning desire to pursue. Although she loved the competition on the university circuit, Olympic qualifying was not a goal.

Since several of her school's coaches were Olympic coaches, this filtered down to mean that the rules of the game were tough for all the wrestlers, and expectations for each team member were at the highest level. Among the many disciplines was to stay tight within predetermined weight classes. This is generally not an easy feat to accomplish. It meant employing the sweating-it-out-methods on a continual basis to "make weight" for matches and to keep coaches happy.

The pressure of making weight to qualify for classes was always stressful, and having Type 1 diabetes compounded Jen's situation. The combination of working out strenuously, sometimes limiting food intake before tournament weigh-ins, and following an intense training schedule does not bode well with maintaining good or even decent diabetes control. Jen found it nearly impossible to handle these stresses, but being the passionate sport and team player that she is, she worked hard at trying to manage both for thirteen years. During wrestling season a typical week would go something like this:

- one team practice and one partner training session daily totaling
- three hours fitness and weight training
- weekend tournaments and competitions

Breaking the Mold
Generally speaking, wrestling is a male dominated sport. When Jen started out, she didn't know any other girls who had even heard of women's wrestling, let alone participated in the sport. It is quite different today, however, with over 6000 young women competing in collegiate wrestling in the United States alone, as part of the Women's College Wrestling Association.

In 2004, women's wrestling was the only new sport introduced at the Olympic Games in Athens. Fifty-four nations were represented in the sport at those games, and one of Jen's teammates (who eventually became her varsity coach at Brock University), Tonya Verbeek, won silver in Athens. This was beyond exciting and a cause for celebration for Jen's team and the entire Canadian wrestling community.

One-to-one combat is not new to women. Its history can be traced back as far as the fifteenth century with brawls, dueling and martial arts. In the U.S., the 1950s, '60s and '70s were the golden age of ladies professional freestyle and Greco-Roman wrestling. Beverly "The Hammer" Shade and Natasha "The Hatchet Lady" were two of the well known professional wrestlers of the day. Wrestling still conjures rough-and-tumble bawdiness to a degree, but in fact it has become a sport of athletic prowess and discipline. The Mat (*www.themat.com*), the Canadian Wrestling Association (*www.wrestling.ca*), NCAA (*www.ncaa.com*) and the Canadian Saskatchewan (*www.saskwrestling.com*) have detailed information for those interested in knowing more about the sport.

On both the high school "scholastic" and university "freestyle" levels, Jen trained with boys. For matches and competitions, the sexes were separated. In the U.S., "folk-style" university wrestling is practiced with an entirely different set of rules. Jen found that training with the boys motivated her to be the best she could. She enjoyed the fact that in training everyone viewed each other as athletes, disregarding gender. Wrestling has changed over the years and there has been rapid growth in the sport, especially among females and mixed gender competition. As Jen notes:

I had teammates who were actively working toward the goal of winning an Olympic medal, something that was not possible five years ago. I had one teammate who achieved the ultimate goal and won both silver and bronze medals at the Olympic Games.

Jen believes there is merit to inspiring by example. Seeing women such as her perform and compete in a sport like wrestling is surely a profound motivator to other women with diabetes.

I asked Jen if diabetes played any role in her decision to wrestle. "Having diabetes didn't influence my decision to wrestle, but it taught me to be more in tune with my body and health," she said.

Jen's Strategy

Wrestling is an action-reaction sport. For the most part, Jen was a defensive wrestler and tried to learn all she could about her opponents' strategies before going to the mat. Jen told me that she spent lots of time studying her opponents before matches. This strategy gave her some insight of what to expect when an offensive opponent went after her with a double leg takedown or half nelson or throw. In case you don't know about ladies wrestling moves and what it takes to win a match, here's a brief rundown:

Winning a match can be achieved by:

- Pinning an opponent's shoulders on the mat for a count of two seconds
- Dominating to a point of technological superiority
- Default
- Disqualification by illegal or rough moves

Legal Moves: Olympic freestyle wrestling has many rules that insure that no trained wrestler is at risk of being badly injured. Throws such as the hip toss, fireman's carry and shoulder throw are a few of the legal moves. Other strategies include pinning moves and point accumulation.

The Varsity Years

Jen remembers her greatest success during her first year of participation as a varsity athlete. She had her best finish at the national wrestling competition known as the CIS or Canadian Inter-University Sport Championships. Her overall fourth-place finish was something to be proud of. In the Provincial Championship tournaments, Jen placed second, only losing to the current World University Championship title holder. That year was thrilling and challenging for Jen, playing her sport in the team "singlet"—a navy blue and white spandex uniform with bold red letters streaming down the side.

Headgear is not mandatory in Canada as it is in the United States, although it is worn by athletes who compete at intense levels to prevent cauliflower ear. Some of Jen's teammates have had to undergo plastic surgery to correct deformation that occurs with this injury. Jen admits to having some ear damage from her years of wrestling because she opted not to wear headgear which was cumbersome and felt uncomfortable. She trusts that nobody notices her ears today.

The weight class for the university championships was fifteen kilos lower than what she usually wrestled at during high school competitions. Accomplishing the tough new weight standards with careful food intake and extra time in the gym was another huge success for Jen. She felt great at the lower weight and was able to move faster during a typical match, which consists of three rounds of two-minute bouts with a thirty-second breather between each bout. The overall success of that year came because, "I was able to strike a balance between my diabetes, my wrestling and the huge challenges associated with my first year of living away from home and starting university."

Life as a varsity athlete held many great advantages besides playing and competing in a sport you love. There was the camaraderie with teammates and the opportunity to meet and become friends with many great athletes. Being part of a team was also helpful in learning discipline, and Jen feels that "having a team that is depending on me, I am always able to push myself a little further. Even though wrestling is an individual sport, it has team aspects also. In many cases the thrill of winning a team title is much more satisfying than winning an individual championship." In Canada there is an understated sense of respect among women wrestlers. "Although there were certain teams we never bonded with," Jen said, "there were many individuals who were grunt and groan combatants on the mat who became close friends."

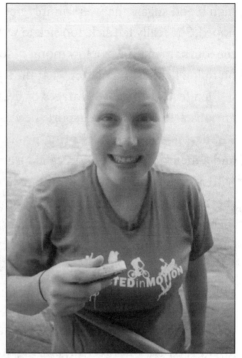

Jen is "Connected In Motion"

Wrestling with Diabetes

While there were many wins during the course of Jen's wrestling career, they were peppered with some disappointments. Managing blood glucose levels, in a sport that requires short bursts of intense anaerobic energy interspersed with brief rest periods, caused her blood glucose levels to fluctuate during many competitions. And, of course, that fear of hypoglycemia which lies hidden in every diabetic's psyche was always there for Jen. *Will I go low?* is the nagging question all of us understand.

High blood sugars are another story. One time at the beginning of her wrestling career, she was scheduled for a qualifying tournament at the provincial championships. Because women's wrestling was still a fairly new sport, there were few girls in the classification. All she was required to do was show up at the tournament to qualify, even if she had to forfeit all of her matches. Jen wasn't feeling well that day due to high blood sugars that were simply not moving down as quickly as she hoped. She really felt sick, too sick to walk over to school to show up for the tournament. It was a low moment for Jen who always prided herself on doing her best no matter what the situation.

Jen feels that the advantages of being a varsity athlete outweighed any obstacle. Through her sport she was able to take advantage of some wonderful volunteer mentoring projects, such as being a coordinator and a mentor for a program called IMPACT, which pairs varsity athletes with at-risk youth in the community. As a youngster with diabetes, she attended Camp Huronda, a Canadian camp for children with diabetes, for eight summers. After that she continued as a staff member for another nine years. The friends she met during Camp Huronda days remain some of her best friends. Her time there had a powerful impact on her life, particularly on the direction she would take in her career as a teacher and educator. Through the camp experience and teaching, Jen has been involved with many diabetes organizations. She has worked as a volunteer, organizing fundraising teams for the Juvenile Diabetes Research Foundation and Canadian Diabetes Association. In 2010, she was part of the first Children With Diabetes—Friends For Life conference in Vancouver, working as part of the leadership team of the entire elementary program, a position she is thrilled and honored to fill.

Being plugged into so many diabetes groups has been extremely positive for Jen. She says:

My attitude towards having diabetes is to use it as an opportunity to teach and learn. I have been able to be part of so many great organizations and made friends with many amazing people because of my diabetes. I enjoy showing people and myself as well, that I can do anything I set my mind to, not just despite diabetes but because of diabetes. No dream is impossible as long as you train for it.

But—and this is a big *but*—Jen Hanson is not your average Type 1 or Type 2, or average anything. Jen is a young woman of tremendous substance who is blessed with the gifts of athletic prowess and determination to do her best at everything she pursues. Optimism and her ability to radiate warmth, along with her contagious sense of encouragement, spark a flame in those around her to also do their best. The qualities Jen possesses are reflected in many ways … her love of trying to make a difference in people's lives, her passion for playing music, savoring the company of good friends and continuing to work on her third university degree with high hopes of one day opening her own outdoor education center and summer camp. In 2012, she was awarded a scholarship to pursue her PhD in education at the University of Ottawa.

Jen is proud to be a role model for others who live with diabetes and encourages them to use it as a positive force. She now lives her life with a certain pride of having diabetes and is proud of the accomplishments she has achieved in her life with it. She enjoys telling people about it.

Jen is the only one in her immediate or extended family who has diabetes, and is thrilled that all family members are active in sports, especially outdoor activities like camping and hiking. Her father continues to play hockey every week and her mom takes fitness classes at the local gym. Jen's father has paddled countless lakes and rivers, and both parents have hiked all along the rugged east coast of Canada. Jen looks up to her parents with great admiration and hopes she will continue to be as active as they are when she gets older and has children of her own.

The Sisterhood of Diabetes is just as proud to have in its fold a young woman, Jen Hanson, who gives all of us the same inspiration that she shines on others. Plus, we now know who to go to if we need to learn some defensive moves. Thanks, Jen! ⁂

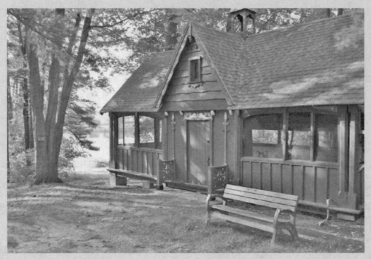

Camp Ho Mita Koda, Newbury, Ohio

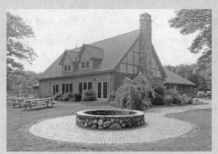

Clara Barton Camp, North Oxford, Massachusetts

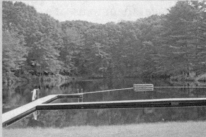

Swimming at Clara Barton Camp

Diabetes Camps

Just a few years after insulin was discovered at the University of Toronto in 1922, and when supplies of insulin were being distributed to physicians with great caution, Dr. Henry John and his wife Betty of Cleveland, Ohio, decided to take six of his patients, young girls with diabetes, to a lake in Newbury, Ohio, where the couple had a summer cottage. Dr. John was the medical personnel for this endeavor while Betty, an avid and accomplished outdoors enthusiast, supervised the activities for the girls. It was an instant success. The following year it became Camp Ho Mita Koda, which means "Welcome My Friend" in the Sioux language. Camp Ho Mita Koda became the first organized diabetes camp in the world, and its mission and high standards continue today without any interruption since that first summer of 1929. Dr. John continued to be active in camp until his passing and his wife Betty did the same until her death in 1997. Today the camp has expanded greatly and is the magical summer home for over three hundred children with diabetes.

Clara Barton (1881-1912), a farm girl from North Oxford, Massachusetts, founded the American Red Cross. Another native of North Oxford, Eliot Joslin (1869-1962), was a renowned physician in the field of childhood diabetes, beginning at a time when insulin had not yet been discovered. After Barton's death, the women's committee of the North Oxford Universalist church, of which Clara had been a member, bought the farmhouse where she was born, restored it as a museum and made use of the land as a summer getaway for inner city kids, a fresh air camp of sorts. Dr. Joslin, the other North Oxford native, approached the church women about joining forces to provide a camp for young girls with diabetes, as a place to improve their health through education, recreation and support programs. The deal was made in 1932 and the camp has never stopped performing its original mission. At that time it was called "The Clara Barton Birthplace Camp" and it opened its doors to serve eight girls the first year. With Dr. Joslin as medical director, it became known as "an island of safety" and "the hospital in the woods." Soon, other diabetes camps opened throughout the country using Clara Barton camp as their model.

In 1948, a brother camp for boys with diabetes, Camp Joslin, opened nearby. Today, The Barton Center for Diabetes Education, Inc. encompasses two resident camps, day camp programs, adventure programs, family camp and a full array of outstanding programming in all seasons to educate and inspire those living with diabetes.   ✂

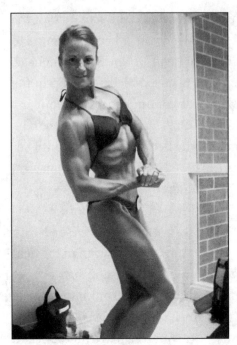

Melissa Prichard

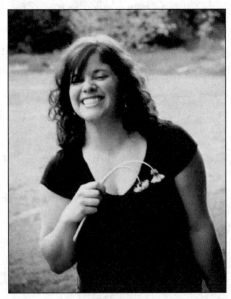

Ginger Vieira

MELISSA PRICHARD AND GINGER VIEIRA

Lifting the Bars

C'mon. Tell the truth. When you hear the term "iron games," which represent bodybuilding, weight lifting and power lifting, do you think of Doug Burns, Mr. Natural Universe and Type 1 diabetic? Or does some other super strong guy come to mind? Or do you think of Type 1 bodybuilder Melissa Prichard and Type 1 power lifter Ginger Vieira? Both women are competitive champions in their respective sports.

To set the record straight on the differences among weight lifting, bodybuilding and power lifting, let's define terms. Weight lifting is an Olympic sport involving speed, skill, flexibility and strength. Power lifting is simply defined as "lifting with power," demonstrating what the muscles can physically achieve. Both have three events which must follow in sequence at competitions: the bench press, the squat and the dead lift. Bodybuilding is the sport of working out with weights to reshape the physique by adding muscle mass and increasing separation and definition of the various muscle groups.

Women's bodies have been the subject of artists' renditions and dictates of the imagination for centuries, going all the way back to the mythological Amazons of ancient Greece. And women pumping iron has intrigued the world in different venues, such as bikini contests in the 1950s and '60s, to women's national physique championships in the '70s, which judged muscularity. Other organizations and competitions followed. They all acted independently until 1980 when the first women's

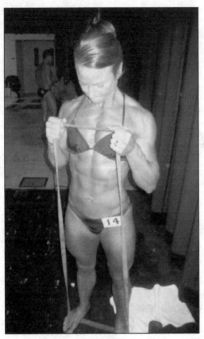

Melissa prepares

national competitions were held and continue today under the auspices of the Federation of Women Body-builders. Bodybuilding came to the public forefront with the movie *Pumping Iron 2: The Women.*

Melissa Prichard

Melissa Prichard participated in sports from the time she was a little girl in Wisconsin. Track and field, volleyball, basketball and other team sports earned her a whopping and record-breaking sixteen varsity letters upon graduation from high school. During a physical examination required for varsity volleyball, at age sixteen, Melissa was diagnosed with Type 1 diabetes. But that didn't stop her from the team sports she loved so, especially basketball.

Melissa's interest in competitive bodybuilding started when her husband recognized her potential. The couple worked out at the gym regularly. One day when he saw Melissa, a great all-around athlete, bench press 160 lbs. with no trouble, he suggested that perhaps it was time to think about entering competitions. So, in early 2008, body-building became her first individual sport.

Being on the stage alone without a team to back her up if something went wrong, sharpened Melissa's sense of competition. She trained and worked diligently not to let anyone down. In August of that same year, she entered her first bodybuilding show at the Wisconsin State Fair where she weighed in at 155 lbs. She won first place in the heavy weight division and second place overall. The victory was a great surprise and boosted her confidence, but she was not sure if she wished to continue with competitions. Bodybuilders are always in training. It takes much time, hard work and dedication. With her career as a registered dietician, Certified Diabetes Educator, and territory manager for Medtronic, plus a family and four dogs, time was a precious commodity. But with the strong encouragement of family and friends she decided to go for it, and still continues to compete in bodybuilding.

Diabetes opened many windows of opportunity for Melissa twenty years ago when she was diagnosed at age sixteen, and has taught her to be both responsible and realistic in life. It has been a driving force in the healthy way she eats and the time she spends exercising. She jokes that she'd like to give it away to any takers, but believes that if it weren't for diabetes, she would be neither a bodybuilder nor diabetes educator.

Melissa is in training for her dream of competing successfully at the national and world levels of bodybuilding, but is proud of what she has achieved so far. She would love to speak out and inspire people with diabetes to challenge their bodies and overcome the diabetes barriers they set for themselves. She knows that we change and challenge our minds, and that we can do the same with our bodies. Melissa has clearly proven this to herself and others. She believes, "We can do anything we want to. Really, we can."

Ginger Vieira

Another strong and powerful young woman who currently holds fifteen records in national federation drug-tested power lifting is Ginger Vieira. Ginger is a twenty-six-year-old Type 1 diabetic diagnosed at age thirteen. This whirlwind of a gal, who was also diagnosed with Celiac Disease at age fourteen, a year after her Type 1 diagnosis, exudes boundless energy and enthusiasm even when she's not bench pressing 190 lbs. Ginger is two-time winner of the Vermont State Bench Press Competition. Bench pressing consists of laying flat on a standardized weight bench while lifting a heavily weighted bar from chest to full arm extension and back, with precision. It is something that must be done with great strength, skill

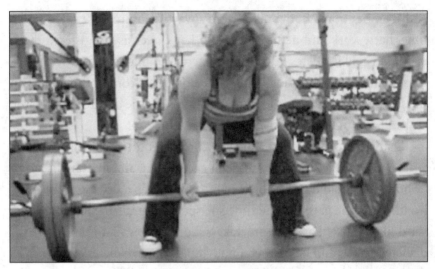

Ginger's power lift

and breathing technique. Besides her record breaking bench press wins, Ginger squats with 265 lbs. of weight and dead lifts over 300 lbs. All of this power and strength comes wrapped in a five-foot-tall frame.

Intense training, hard work and the expert diabetes care it takes to prepare for power lifting competitions is not all that occupies Ginger's time. Ginger has always been athletic and competitive growing up in a household with three brothers who encouraged her to be tough, strong and mainly persistent. Needless to say, she was always the girl in her class who could do the most push-ups and climb the hardest part of the ropes course.

In addition to daily training, Ginger has written several books including *Your Own Diabetes Science Experiments*, based on all she has learned through her own discovery process. Ginger takes the mystery out of high and low blood sugars by explaining the physiological complexities that happen in the body and how to balance them.

When not training or writing her book, Ginger finds time to teach power yoga classes and do cognitive-based coaching, which involves helping her clients use positive coping methods—urging the hard wiring in the brain to build self esteem, manage chronic illnesses, learn new nutrition habits and incorporate exercise in their lives. Ginger also manages to find time to volunteer at a Vermont diabetes summer camp program and to connect with kids as a diabetes mentor.

With so much going on in her life, it is important for Ginger to eat a gluten-free diet because of her Celiac condition. This is not an obstacle to good eating, however, as the Celiac way of eating is quite healthy and wholesome, and based on fresh foods. Gluten-free foods are widely available these days and offer much more variety and availability than they did four years ago. There are even half decent gluten-free pizzas these days.

Ginger believes the "diabetes is a lifelong process" that she keeps learning more about each day. From the looks of things, this accomplished young woman has learned quite a bit already from the process of diabetes.

You can catch up with Ginger's latest findings at:

www.living-in-progress.com
www.twitter.com/gingervieira
www.YouTube.com/usergingervieira
www.healthcentral.com
www.parentingdiabetickids.com

Ginger's diabetes blog, "For Betes Sake" can be found at her website: *www.living-in-progress.com*. She also blogs on *www.diabetesdaily.com*.

To find a local center in your area, as there are no national chains, your best bet is to do a net search for "powerlifting" or "bodybuilding training gyms." You can also locate You Tube videos and a wide variety of websites on these subjects. One example is *www.usapowerlifting.com/newsletter*.

Melissa and Ginger have certainly lifted the bars for all women who aspire to pursue bodybuilding and power lifting. They have also proven that diabetes is not an obstacle to fitness and sports. They are both powerhouses of inspiration in our Sisterhood of Diabetes.   ❦

EMILY CHEUNG
"Call 9-1-1!"

"I consider my first severe low blood sugar to be a defeat in my ability to control my diabetes. It was unexpected, but perhaps caused by jetlag as I had just gotten back to California from a trip to China. I had forgotten to set my alarm and woke up at 2 PM realizing something was wrong. My mind was clear, but my muscles were not reacting to the commands coming from my mind. I got to the phone and dialed my boyfriend at the time. "Mike," I mumbled, "my blood ... sugar's ... low." I realized I was slurring my speech.

"Em, call 9-1-1, I'm coming," Mike said.

I had not thought of calling 9-1-1 myself, perhaps because I didn't think this was a true emergency—I had never been hospitalized for the disease outside of my initial diagnosis. With much concentration I pushed 9...1...1. When the operator came on I forced myself to slowly state, "I'm diabetic, my blood sugar's low. I need sugar." Unfortunately, because there's a triage system to the 9-1-1 line, she transferred me to the paramedic operator who then asked me the same question, and with immense effort I repeated, "I'm diabetic. My blood sugar's low. I need sugar." She asked for my address.

"Can't you get that from caller ID?" I thought, but pointing that out to her would just cost me valuable energy, so I stated my address. She finally confirmed that an ambulance was on its way. I thanked her and dropped the phone.

I was in trouble, big trouble. Throughout my entire life I've been told by diabetes educators, doctors, and others with diabetes to keep sugar by my bedside, but on this day I did not have any there. When my blood sugar is low, I generally like to get orange juice from the refrigerator. Never did I imagine I might be incapacitated to the point where I could not *get* to the refrigerator. Then I remembered that I put *Gu* on my little kitchen console where I put my keys. I normally grabbed it on my way out for a run or workout, but today it would serve a much more urgent purpose.

Unable to walk, I challenged myself, "Emily, you *must* get to the kitchen for this sugar." Then, I crawled there … and finally sat myself in front of the console. To my right was the front door of my house. In one jerky motion I moved my right arm up to grab a *Gu* packet and then just stared at it, unable to open the package. I knew that I needed to open it, for *my life*, and I just couldn't!

"Emily, focus! You will not pass out! You have to open this *Gu*," I told myself. It took every brain cell I had to figure out how. I ended up ripping the top off with my left hand, while my right hand held and squirted the packet. Because my hand muscles were not working properly, the first squirt spilled on my leg, but I managed to get the second mouthful. I felt some mental relief knowing that the sugar should prevent me from passing out, still, it would take time to absorb.

My front door was locked, but I could not get myself up to reach it. As I sat there the paramedics arrived. "Ma'am, you need to open this door," they called.

"Yes, I know," I said in very slurred speech. But I couldn't. Again they asked me to open the door. This time I looked at the lock and used my last ounce of strength to get to it and turn the knob to open. Compared to the Paris Marathon, this felt harder, lots harder, like that was the last of everything I had in me. [See her story page 142.]

Once inside, the paramedics kindly told me everything would be okay and checked my blood sugar. One paramedic started IV dextrose and then prepared me for transfer to the Emergency Dept. (ED).

Once discharged from the ED, however, I soon experienced two more severe low blood sugar episodes. It was time for me to have a better monitoring system in place to detect and prevent going low. So I filled out appropriate papers and submitted them to my health plan to approve a Continuous Glucose Monitor (CGM).

The first denial came from a health plan endocrinologist. I appealed the decision and two administrative reviews were held. Again denied! I felt ashamed for requesting a machine that two panels of experts had ruled I did not need.

Through the help of a friend, however, I accessed a second opinion at an academic hospital and the case escalated to the California State Department for Independent Medical Review. Finally, the state reviewer overturned previous denials and supported my request for the CGM. My persistence paid off.

Even though it takes time and energy, perseverance usually wins—whether training for a marathon or working through the steps for medical system appeals. With the continued support of my boyfriend and family and friends I am doing very well with my CGM and blood glucose trends. Since my initial challenges in obtaining the device, research has been published sanctioning its many benefits for diabetic patients.

CHAPTER 5

Exploring Life's Summit

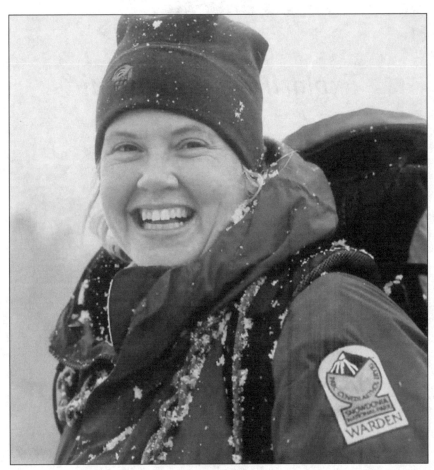

Nikki Wallis

NIKKI WALLIS

Climbing Her Way with Diabetes, Music and Many Mountains

Now here's an adventure story for you that involves a Type 1 athlete. Nikki Wallis is a mountaineer. She is part of the Snowdonia National Park's rescue squad. Snowdonia Mountain is the highest peak in North Wales. Locals call it "The Burial Place." Legend has it that dragons, giants and even King Arthur himself perished in this merciless mountain. Some say that the good king's sword, Excalibur, hides in Snowdonia Mountain.

One day a few years ago, Nikki, a member of the Snowdonia Rescue Squad since an early age, was making her rounds on the mountain with Jakob, her rescue dog companion. It was 3:30 in the afternoon and she expected to be down the mountain by 5:30 when darkness and an approaching storm bringing ice, snow and frozen trails would creep in. As they patrolled the mountain, Nikki heard a faint sound in the distance. It was probably wind gathering in the crevasses and flanks of the mountain due to the gathering storm, she thought. But when the sound repeated, she realized it was not the wind. With Jakob leading the way to test the uneven ground, they moved along a narrow ragged trail towards the faint sound. Soon it became clear that it was a cry for help.

As Nikki eventually made her way to the source of the voice, she spotted two young climbers clinging with their hands to a dangerous icy incline on the edge of a cliff. Directly below them was an eight-hundred feet drop. One of the climbers was slipping.

Immediately Nikki calculated their location with her compass and map, and radioed the ranger station for help. She struggled to carry and coax the endangered climbers to relative safety, made a cover for them with the Mylar tent she carried in her backpack, and soon both the climbers, along with Nikki and Jakob, were huddled for warmth as they waited for the rescue squad to reach them. Their location was not accessible by helicopter, which meant the rescuers would have to climb their way, in the dark, up the narrow and now icy and treacherous path to find the distressed climbers. Nikki, who has Type 1 diabetes, began to worry that her blood sugar might start dropping since her plan had been to be down the mountain by 5:30 when darkness set in. With half a cheese and jam sandwich and some sugar cubes buried in her pack, she knew she had to keep the two climbers awake and alert, and if possible nourished, until the rescue squad arrived.

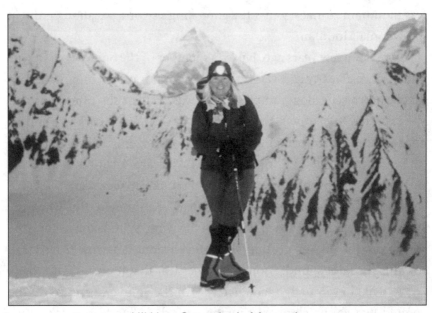

Nikki on Snowdonia Mountain

Weather conditions were worsening by the minute. Nikki wished she had her flute (or piano) handy since she is an accomplished classical musician. She would play beautiful music for them. Instead, with a smile she began to tell the boys stories and legends about the mountain and anything else she could think of.

The young climbers told her that they had intended merely a nice walk in the mountains to enjoy the view. One of them had never climbed before and both wore only sneakers. All they carried with them was a bag of chips and books to read on the mountain. Meanwhile, Nikki periodically stuck her head outside the makeshift shelter to wave her high beam flashlight in hopes that the rescuers would soon find them. One of the boys had fallen one hundred feet down a cliff and his knee was in very bad shape. She performed first aid on him but he would obviously need a lot more than this.

At 11:30 PM, after sixteen hours on the mountain, Nikki heard the welcome voices of the rescue team. Her directions had been perfect but the trail was most difficult. They secured the injured climber onto a stretcher, while the other young man was carried on the back of a rescuer. Nikki, the only female ranger in Snowdonia Park, walked the two-hour trek down the mountain with her dog Jakob and her husband, Neil Rawlinson, also a member of the Snowdonia Rescue Squad, who had made his way onto the mountain to accompany her down. Once on firm ground she was fine—weary, tired and thirsty— but fine. Her blood sugar had been fully cooperative throughout the long and sometimes stressful day. When she finally got home to an open fire, some food and a glass of red wine, she soon dozed off into a deep sleep.

The next morning, newspapers throughout the United Kingdom headlined Nikki and Jakob as "The Snowdonia Blizzard Heroes." Certainly it had been an adventure but, as Nikki said, "It's part of the job as a member of the mountain rescue squad."

A Few Things About Nikki

Nikki Wallis was born in a small village in the mountains of North Wales, and though she has travelled and lived in many locations, including the mountains of South Africa, Snowdonia is always home. Along with her brother Craig, she began climbing when she was a wee four years old. Her parents were excellent mountaineers. Her father was a UIAGM (Union Internationale des Associations de Guides de Montagnes) mountain guide, and her mom was one of the first women to qualify for outdoor mountain leader walking certification. Nikki grew up a tomboy, roughing it up in the mud on the football field and playing hockey at school. She loved swimming and biking, but walking in the mountains was where she belonged. She and her brother explored treacherous sailing and mountaineering expeditions from an early age.

As a teenager, Nikki ventured out on her own into the mountains and became absorbed in nature and the outdoor environment. In 1984, she took a rock climbing course with an internationally renowned mountain guide, Brede Arkless. This course inspired Nikki to try her skills on indoor rock-climbing walls, where she realized that she had good balance and flexibility, and was prepared to climb difficult trails in the mountains.

As she explored the mountains of Snowdonia, Nikki acquired or sharpened many other survival skills—including her instinct, her knowledge of weather, and abilities in map reading, an important key to safe mountaineering. At age seventeen, Nikki applied for a spot on the local mountain rescue team, but instead made the decision to tend to her studies at the University in Sheffield first, before dedicating herself to full-time mountain rescue work.

Climbing with Diabetes

Nikki spent the summer of her twenty-fourth year rock climbing in Yosemite Valley, California. This was quite an exciting time with many terrific challenges. When she returned to Wales, and with an undergraduate degree in Biochemistry and Molecular Biology, she embarked on a post-graduate teacher certification course in Outdoor Pursuits and Science. Shortly after she began her graduate studies, however, she had an incident of falling and passing out in her backyard garden as she was taking in wash from the clothes line. Her (former) husband's rescue dog found her and alerted her husband. She was taken to the hospital and released later that night with a diagnosis of a concussion. But something else was not right. She felt awful and her condition worsened. She went back to the hospital several days later where they performed numerous investigative tests. One morning during the hospital stay a nurse walked into Nikki's room carrying a tray that contained an orange-colored syringe and vial of insulin. She was told, matter- of-factly, that she had Type 1 diabetes, and instructed that she would have to inject insulin on a daily basis from that day forward.

How could this be? Nikki Wallis, healthy mountaineer and rescue squad member, rock climber, athlete. It just didn't seem right.

Nikki had quite a struggle to accept the reality of diabetes at first. Sixteen years ago in North Wales, no information was available on the interplay of diabetes and mountaineering. In fact, no information existed *anywhere*. This was a challenge unlike anything she was used to, and Nikki knew she needed to dig in with her psychological crampons and master this new mountain.

It took a while, but Nikki found the strength and determination to adapt a positive mindset and deal with diabetes. She knew she was not going to stop her outdoor life and so she needed to learn everything she could about diabetes and sports, particularly about managing diabetes and mountains, which she did. Through many trial and error experiments, Nikki learned to coordinate necessary diabetes skills such as advanced planning and predicting situations into her mountaineering.

One day, the floodgates of possibility opened for her when Nikki learned of a mountain climber with Type 1 diabetes who had scaled Mt. Gasherbrum in the Himalayas. This moved her into first gear to establish a support group for adventurous diabetics. In 2000, she formed Mountains for Active Diabetics (MAD). Over the years the group has grown internationally to engage in adventurous outdoor pursuits. They have become a renowned resource of expert individuals who instruct in managing diabetes in remote and hostile expedition settings. MAD constantly seeks better diabetes management while engaging in challenging outdoor adventures.

More Adventurous Pursuits

Athletes who live with diabetes often seek out and attract others of like mind. They form a beautiful tapestry woven with care, support, challenges, knowledge, inspiration and enthusiasm. Always read for new challenges, Nikki frequently speaks to a wide variety of groups addressing the discrimination that often exists about diabetes. She portrays a different image of people with diabetes by exemplifying some of the incredible adventures and challenges she has seen and faced. Currently, Nikki is studying for her nursing degree with the intention of working in the field of emergency care and diabetes. Her studies have made her acutely aware of how serious complications surrounding diabetes can arise, and how frightening they can be. It has also made her mindful of the importance of keeping life and diabetes in balance and perspective while seeking out new pursuits.

Another interest Nikki has been engaging in for a few years now is long distance mountain-lake swimming. While in Montana for a MADIDEA 2007 gathering, a group of fellow diabetic mountaineers, including David Panofsky, Doug Bursnall, Jeff Mazer and Mauro Surmani, decided to swim a high altitude lake (8,500 ft.) at the base camp of Mount Cowen. Since then Nikki frequently swims 2K in a local pool to strengthen her freestyle stroke in preparation for accomplishing her goal to swim as many outdoor lakes as possible all over the world. Nikki is of the mindset that experimental playing or performing in the sport and *training* for a sport is the same.

Spare Time?

Music is a gift that Nikki embraces passionately—she enjoys playing both piano and flute, along with teaching students in these instruments. Being the proud and indulgent auntie of her brother's triplet daughters who live in Australia is another great joy for her. Sitting down at the end of a busy day, enjoying some freshly made guacamole with chips and a glass of red wine soothes her body and spirit and encourages her to dream of future projects and initiatives, and about making a difference in the lives of people with diabetes.

Nikki sometimes recalls a famous quote from W.H. Murray, Scottish mountaineer and writer:

> *Until committed there is hesitancy, the chance to draw back, always ineffectiveness. Concerning all acts of initiative and creation there is one elementary truth, the ignorance of which kills countless ideas and splendid plans: that the moment one definitely commits oneself, then Providence moves, too. All sort of things occur to help one that would never otherwise have occurred. A whole stream of events issues from the decision, raising in one's favor all matter of unforeseen incidents and meetings and material assistance, which no man could have dreamt would have come his way. I have learned a deep respect for one of Goethe's couplets—*

> *Whatever you can do, or dream you can, begin it.*
> *Boldness has genius, power and magic in it.*

Here is a short list of some information about Nikki Wallis:

- UK Mountain Leader Qualified *www.mlte.org*
- Himalayan mountain climber (Karakorum and Pamirs)
- Rock climber and mountaineer for over twenty years
- Mountain biker and Sponsored Diabetic Triathlete

- National Park Ranger for 9+ years *www.snowdonia-npa.org.uk*
- Founder of Mountains for Active Diabetics *www.mountain-mad.org*
- Winner of DESA Athletic Achievement Award 2005 *www.diabetes-exercise.org*
- Runner up of Diabetes UK "contribution to diabetes" HG Wells Award
- Profiled athlete in Dr. Sheri Colberg Ochs *Diabetic Athletes Handbook 2009*
- Coach-U trained
- Professional international lecturer on practical management of diabetes for many courses and medical groups
- Professional member of Diabetes UK
- Active member of local mountain rescue team
- Retired Chairperson and SAR dog handler in the Search and Rescue Dog Association
- Passionate about bridging the information gap enabling individuals to proactively manage their diabetes in the mountains

I had the privilege to meet Nikki and her mom in 2007 at Westchester University in Pennsylvania when Nikki was awarded the LifeScan Athletic Achievement Award. I felt an immediate bond with both these women because of our common Welch heritage (I'm a Jones). And now there is the powerful bond of the Sisterhood of Diabetes that Nikki's strength and zest for life shares with all of us.

Thanks, Nikki for getting us up the mountain.   🦋

HEIDI-JANE HUMPHRIES

From First 10k at One Year Old to Multiple Ironman Victories

Near her home in Christchurch, New Zealand, Heidi-Jane ran her first 10k race from a jogging stroller that her father pushed when she was just one year old. She loved watching the fast runners from her comfortable little perch. It may have sparked something in this youngster because she started running track and cross country by the time she was seven. At ten she was doing middle distance runs and winning races.

In 2007 at age twenty-nine, Heidi-Jane placed sixth in the ITU (International Triathlon Union). She then joined the World Duathlon Championship, which consists of a 10k run, followed by a 40k cycle and then a 5k run. In 2008, she completed her first Ironman in 11 hours 51 minutes. She hasn't stopped competing in these challenging races that she is so passionate about and she is still proud and thrilled to hear

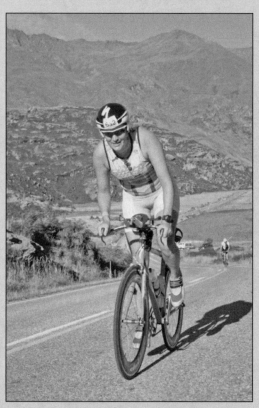

Heidi-Jane Humphries

Diabetes Pet Peeves?

The things that bothered "Ironman" Heidi-Jane Humphries the most were when people who didn't understand anything about diabetes would make comments like, "Oh, you must have a really severe case of diabetes because of all the insulin you take." She also hated it when folks compared her to their obese Type 2 uncle.

Those of us with diabetes all have our pet peeves—a long list for some—and they can drive us bonkers. What are yours?

I remember being at a diabetes and sports conference in Mission Springs, California, where one stormy night about fifty of us were cooped up in a small cabin. We started going around the room citing "diabetes pet peeves." At first we were angry and disgusted but at a certain point we began to laugh and make light of our common plight. Humor can be great medicine.

the words that hooked her when she crossed the finish line of her first Ironman: "Heidi-Jane Humphries you are an Ironman."

In working to raise awareness and management of diabetes, she has set up a charity in New Zealand called "T1 Consulting." Its main focus is assisting people with Type 1 diabetes to take part in sports and exercise safely. Heidi-Jane and her husband Mark have created opportunities for teams of runners, cyclists and triathletes to participate in various events around New Zealand together.

Since the first Ironman in 2008, Heidi-Jane has competed in Ironman NZ 2010, Ironman NZ 2011 and ChallengeWanaka 2012 (also an Ironman event). She has won several marathons and half-marathons and raced in three-day cycle tours. We in the Sisterhood of Diabetes thank you, Heidi-Jane, for enlightening and inspiring us to go for the gold and not be deterred. We are so proud to have you on our side. ✆

CHAPTER 6

Moving With All Types

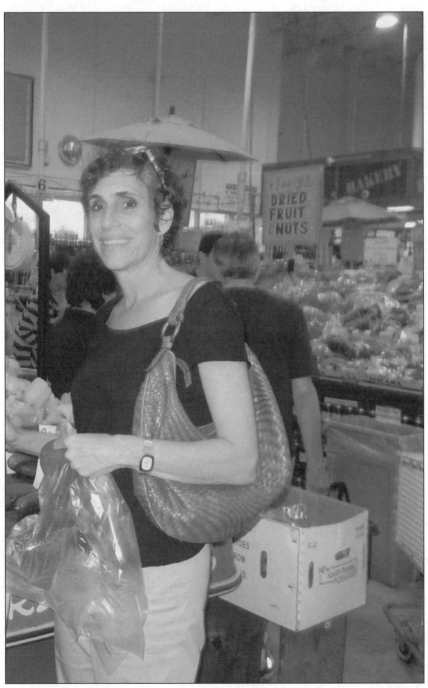

Audrey Finkelstein

AUDREY FINKELSTEIN

Mover and Shaker in the Diabetes Community

The streets and stoops of Brooklyn in the 1950s and '60s were magical places to play and grow up in. Neighborhood kids met after school to run around and play stickball and games like ringalevio and charades. They rode bicycles, double-Dutched jumprope and fastened roller skates on their shoes to race around the block. Playing in the street was safe for kids back then. It was a time when a Spalding ball, some marbles and choosing sides in snowball fights created fun; when neighborhood mothers stuck their heads out the window if they heard kids fighting, and one loud shout to "Stop it" always worked; when imaginations soared, and neighborhoods held block parties with homemade food and fireworks in July. It was a time that molded character and taught life lessons. For those of us from that generation it holds nostalgic memories. Audrey Finkelstein was one of those kids who grew up on a stoop in Brooklyn.

Through education, hard work and a dash of chutzpah, Audrey grew into a highly respected teacher, a dynamic sales rep, and a powerhouse in the international diabetes community. After graduation from Lincoln High School in Brooklyn and Baruch College in New York City, she taught business in a tough school in one of the toughest neighborhoods in the city, the Crown Heights section of Brooklyn. After working as a teacher for four years and as department head for two years, Audrey felt it was time for her to switch gears and expand her life into the business world. She applied for a job with a medical device company, was hired as a sales rep, and soon was promoted to trainer, which meant training the company's sales force. She had found her niche in this area of the business world and flourished in it. While working for a company that produced IV pumps, she met her "perfect compliment" future husband, Walter, and their partnership continues to flourish today. One of the great joys of their marriage is their daughter Becky, who is currently in law school.

Entry to the Diabetes World

In 1998, Audrey went to work for a small new company, the Animas Corporation. Its main focus then was to develop a diabetes tool that would read blood glucose levels on a continuous basis. Today this type of tool is, of course, known as a continuous glucose monitor or CGM. Animas realized that in order to "close the loop" between a continuous monitoring system and insulin delivery, they would need an insulin pump. So, while they were still developing the continuous sensor, they began to develop the R-1000 pump, which was launched in 2000.

Audrey's job with Animas had been as vice president of marketing, customer service and clinical affairs. With the advent of the pump division, she added sales to the job description as well. Her outstanding abilities to market and sell products, as well as connect with people on a deep level of compassion and warmth, made her a natural for the job. Maybe it is her Brooklyn "gut" that enables her to choose the right people for the job—people who are passionate, caring and understanding. Animas was Audrey's introduction to the diabetes world and it became a rewarding place for her to nourish and be nourished for many years.

Audrey Finkelstein is a power magnet who instinctually knows her way around peoples' feelings. (Perhaps that's something else learned on the stoops of Brooklyn.) When Audrey meets someone, no matter who they are, the question always comes to mind: "What does this person need to make their life and the lives of all in the diabetes community better?" Once she understands those needs, she sets out like a whirling dervish to help accomplish worthy goals, both as a leader and a team player. Through her position and networks, Audrey has become an ambassador for the diabetes community. Through her business acumen, she has been able to accomplish so many positive and innovative changes.

Devotion

One of the great loves in Audrey's life is CWD, Children With Diabetes. She travels to their conferences and jumps right in as a volunteer wherever she is needed, whether it be checking off names at the registration desk, or singing songs and cuddling the little toddler groups. She loves the little ones, and being with them reminds her of when her own

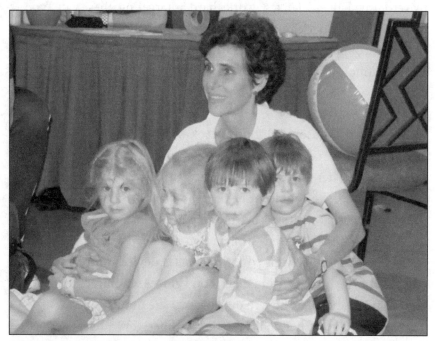

A tender moment: Audrey and her toddlers

daughter Becky was a toddler. Becky now volunteers at CWD also, as does Audrey's husband Walter Greenfield who distributes T-shirts, gives people directions and chats with parents. The Finkelstein-Greenfields are a family of commitment and devotion to helping those in need. Seeing the kids happy and the parents realize that there can be a good life with diabetes is a great boost for each of them.

Audrey recalls how the organization of CWD all began with the passion of a father (Jeff Hitchcock), whose young daughter Marissa was diagnosed with Type 1 diabetes, and a mother (Laura Billedeux), whose son Sam had the same diagnosis. Children With Diabetes has grown to become an international organization serving thousands of families with diabetes. As Audrey says, "Never underestimate the power of parents whose children have diabetes."

Audrey is also involved as a board member with the non-profit "Put Up Your Dukes" organization, begun by former professional football player Jamie Dukes. "Dukes" works hard at targeting obesity in Type 2s in the African-American community. Audrey also sits on the corporate board of Congresso, a grassroots organization dedicated to the under-served Latino community in North Philadelphia.

Her Own Diabetes

In 2006 when Johnson & Johnson took over Animas Corporation, all executives were required to undergo a complete physical examination. Much to her surprise Audrey had a high blood sugar reading. In panic mode, she could not believe the diagnosis, but decided to be super compliant. She tested her blood glucose many times a day, until her fingers became bruised, swollen and ached with pain, right down to the bone. Since she worked for a diabetes device company and had witnessed many people using their blood glucose monitors to test their blood sugars, she knew how to do it—or so she thought.

One day, one of her colleagues noticed her gory fingers and asked her to do a check in front of him. What he immediately noticed was that

Audrey had been piercing her fingers with a raw or uncapped lancing device. Ouch! She learned something new that day.

MODY

Maturity-onset Diabetes of Youth, also called MODY, is a type of diabetes that was named in 1964. It referred to youth who had persistent asymptomatic hyperglycemia without progression to ketoacidosis. By 1990, understanding of MODY became more refined. It is a type of monogeneic diabetes inherited from a parent from one of a small pool of approximately nine genes, and refers to ineffective insulin production or release of pancreatic beta cells. Type 1 and Type 2 are caused from a much larger pool of genes or other factors. MODY is the final diagnosis of 1-2 percent of people diagnosed with diabetes. When first given its name, it appeared to occur in youth up to age twenty, but more recent research shows that it can be diagnosed up to fifty years of age.

A diagnosis of MODY can fall through the cracks. So, how does one know if they have MODY? The most accurate diagnosis can only be determined by extensive and expensive genetic testing. Of the nine genes known to cause MODY, there are tests available for six of them. Since symptoms are the same as in Type 1 and Type 2, diagnosis by any other means can only be suspected. If it is clear that the patient's condition is in fact MODY, treatment recommendations vary from oral hypoglycemic agents to insulin. Other recommendations for successful treatment are:

1. Good glycemic control (as in all cases of diabetes)
2. Regular home checking of blood sugars
3. Healthy meals
4. Physical activity

Her Type 2 diagnosis, after some additional testing, was changed to Mature Onset diabetes in Youth, known as MODY. She treats her condition with a healthy low carbohydrate diet and daily exercise. Maybe she doesn't play stickball in the street anymore or clamp on roller skates the way she did back in Brooklyn, but she power walks four miles a day, takes Zumba classes, does weight training, and works with a trainer at the gym to stay fit and toned and to keep her diabetes condition at bay. By checking her blood sugars, she *knows* that exercise really does have a profound effect on the numbers. And, as Audrey says, "Being pro-active is not only good for maintaining a healthy toned body, it is good for emotional health as well."

Anyone who gets a chance to meet Audrey Finkelstein and be in her presence walks away with a sprinkling of wisdom, warmth and positive energy. She inspires you with a new excitement to be your best in your own path of life.

Our pathways meander and change throughout our lives and Audrey likes to quote Dr. Seuss on this subject saying, "Don't be sorry it's over, be glad it happened." She dreams that one day she will attend Friends of Life conferences for children with diabetes when it is simply Friends For Life and no more diabetes. And so, we are privileged to have Audrey Finkelstein as a friend for life among us in the Sisterhood of Diabetes.

ROSE SCOVEL

Run Like Hell with Type 2

In the midst of planning the young adult Halloween party for St. Paul's Church in Indianapolis, Rose Scovel's great friend and college roommate, Kara, who happens to be a tri-athlete, offered Rose a proposal, more like a challenge—to enter the upcoming Indianapolis Halloween-costume 3-mile race with her. Its theme—"Run Like Hell."

It surely *would be* a challenge, Rose thought, unsure that she could actually make it to the end. But, she accepted! And, much to her own amazement, she accomplished it. Dressed as Neo from "The Matrix," Rose nearly flew across the finish line in fifty minutes … and not quite in the back of the pack.

This Halloween run took place only a few months after Rose was diagnosed with Type 2 diabetes in August 2008. The diagnosis followed a routine medical checkup, and showed an elevated blood glucose level. The doctor ordered a glucose tolerance test.

After the test, Rose felt dreadfully ill for the remainder of the day. Two days later she was notified that the results gave evidence of Type 2 diabetes, and that her A1C was a very high level 9.4. In a strange way she almost expected it, since Type 2 diabetes runs in her family. But she wasn't ready for it to appear on the scene when she was just thirty-two years old. She was scared and knew that she must change her non-exercise lifestyle. It was time for "the fat chick—who made jokes that I wouldn't run unless a really scary man was chasing me, even then I'd

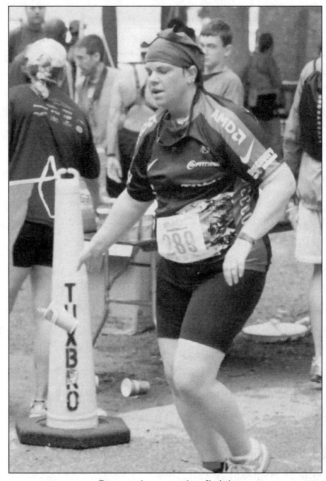

Rose, close to the finish

have to think twice about running"—to change her attitude about exercise. And that happened at the Halloween run.

Maybe simply being with her best friend, or the thrill of being part of a race, or the costume itself did it. It could have been facing the challenge of diabetes that motivated Rose. No matter what the reason was, as she puts it, "I got off my butt and became more active and much healthier." Rose was hooked on running races the minute she crossed the finish line in "Run Like Hell."

Next came the "Drumstick Dash," a tough 4.5 mile Thanksgiving run. She was a little nervous about this one since she had been experiencing low mid-morning blood sugars at that time. She rallied her two sisters to enter the race with her, which they did. That race was a little rough going, but once again Rose crossed the finish line.

In December, she signed up for the "Jingle Bell" run and finished once again. After that run she had another A1C blood test. The results showed that her number had dropped to 6.5 from the original 9.4 reading. Rose Scovel was on her merry way to managing her diabetes with exercise with a sport she enjoyed participating in. She was becoming a runner.

A new incentive came with the Indianapolis Mini-Marathon, which she signed on for to help motivate another friend to run. The Indy Mini is the world's largest half-marathon, the real deal ... without a fun theme and without a costume. Rose knew that this was a serious race and she was about to cross the line! She would have to step up her training for this contest of fleetness.

To prepare herself and help achieve this goal, she acquiesced to her penchant for theme runs and ran the 3-mile New Year's Day "Resolution Revolution" followed by the "Polar Bear" run in February and the "Shamrock Run" in March. She ran the "ADA Race to the Cure" in April, as well as a 15K training run which she managed to finish with a 15:12 pace.

Rose crossed the finish line in the Indianapolis Mini in 3:19:34 and raised $1,000 for the National Youth for Christ Juvenile Justice Ministries.

From Feet to Pedals to Swim Fins

With her incentive bubbling, Rose was ready to take on a new curiosity—cycling. After all, the American Diabetes Association Tour de Cure was coming up in June. It was time to dust off the bicycle she conveniently had not noticed sitting in the back of the garage for over four years. During training for the Tour de Cure, she discovered that she really enjoyed cycling. The morning of the ride, at the last minute, something wild happened. Rose changed her registration program. Instead of entering the 10-mile track ride, she decided to go all out for the 35K road ride. She successfully finished that race with a great sense of accomplishment.

Soon after that ride, her husband David surprised her with a brand new shiny road bike, which inspired additional motivation in Rose. And to top off the victory, her next A1C was an outstanding 5.8! It seemed that all her efforts and dedication to exercise were paying off handsomely.

Pretty soon, Kara the triathlete began teasing her friend Rose about entering a triathlon. After all, Rose had proven herself as a runner and cyclist, and as for the swimming … well, she *had* taken swim classes as a child, up until high school. A triathlon would certainly be a "testing limits" encounter. Rose thought about this new challenge for a while and then called Kara. "Game on," she announced to her friend.

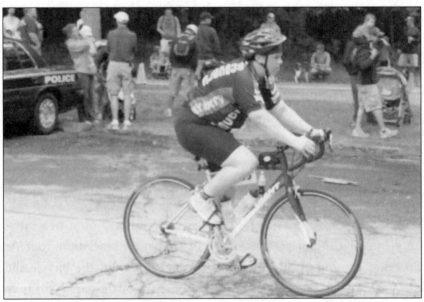

Rose Scovel, tri-athlete

Rose had a couple of months to train and practice swimming for the "Go Girl" triathlon. She joined a community center pool and jumped in the water—her first time swimming in ten years! Understandably she was pretty rusty at first, but knew that she had to do it if she was going to finish the triathlon in less than two hours.

Rose remembered how much she loved swimming during her teenage years and tried to bring that into her practice. When August and the "Go Girl" triathlon came, Rose's determination and discipline paid off. She crossed the finish line in 1:56:45.

Time for the Big One

Rose had taken on some additional gutsy challenges as she trained for the "Go Girl." In July she rode her first 50-mile bike ride, and entered a Personal Best 5-mile run. She was on a roll now—entering, improving and finishing runs, bike races and swim events.

If you guessed that running a marathon would be the next challenge this "non-athlete" would accept, you would have guessed right. As my friend, Type 1 marathoner, Bill King always says in his lectures on diabetes and being active, "We are all athletes. It's up to you to find the athlete within yourself." Rose Scovel had discovered and motivated the athlete within herself with great joy and satisfaction. She signed up for the Indianapolis Monumental Marathon.

Training for this event took her to 15K and 30K races. She finished last in the 30K, but had a good run until the final few miles. Her time for that race was 4:34:14. Shortly after, she walked the 5K AIDS Walk DC in 39:57 minutes—a major achievement for her. Now she was training for a 26.5 run—a marathon!

At mile-marker eleven of the Indianapolis Monumental Marathon, Rose suddenly felt ill. She struggled to keep up her pace for as long as she physically could, but by mile fifteen she knew she needed to stop running, and she dropped out of the race. Sometimes life sprinkles raindrops on our parade. But in Rose's case, as soon as the rain stopped she was back on track training and racing. She ran thirteen half-marathons and rode in the annual RAGBRAI [Register's Annual Great Bike Ride Across Iowa]. She completed three sprint triathlons in 2010, and even attempted her first Olympic distance triathlon along the way. (While she finished the swim and bike parts, unforeseen nutrition problems forced her to drop out for the run. Since then, a sports nutritionist has helped her with both her diabetes and proper nutrition for the endurance sports she participates in.)

And then it happened! Rose finished the San Diego Rock 'n Roll Marathon in June 2011 in 7:09:25. What a day! Motivated by this accomplishment, she plans to give the Indianapolis Monumental Marathon another try. This time her goal is to cross the finish line within 6:30. My money is definitely with Rose on this challenge. She also looks forward to giving the Olympic triathlon another try.

It is quite remarkable to think that someone who entered a fun run called "Run Like Hell" in 2088 had now completed more than eighty races including nineteen half-marathons. The expression "You go, girl" really has meaning when it comes to our Rose Scovel.

Another Platform

Living with the unexpected timing of Rose's Type 2 diabetes diagnosis has proven to be a major motivating factor in her now highly active lifestyle. Although at first she did not want anyone to know about her diabetes, these days she says, "I think having diabetes sucks, but at the same time it is probably one of the best things that happened to me."

Once she got her footing on living with Type 2 diabetes, Rose became an advocate for education and awareness for people under the age of sixty-five diagnosed with this condition. In addition, she hopes to see a decrease of childhood Type 2. National Institute of Health and American Diabetes Association statistics show that instances of Type 2 diabetes in children are growing. The minority groups that have the most substantial increases are the Asian and the Pacific Islanders.

Proportions in African-American and Hispanic groups are about equal to Caucasians. Overweight due to poor diet and sedentary lifestyle is the culprit.

Rose has a list of messages to send out to everyone regarding Type 2 diabetes:

- Type 2 diabetes isn't a social disease brought on just by lifestyle.
- You can live well and have fun while still having diabetes.
- We all need to adopt healthier lifestyles.
- The way our communities develop and function is a part of promoting healthier lifestyles.

Rose's passion about diabetes makes her a powerful a role model and inspiration when she talks about women with diabetes being more visible, especially the younger, under-fifty group. She wants to see Team Type 1 and Team Type 2 cycle groups for women. She wants to see all the faces of diabetes, from little children to the elderly, on TV and in magazines to show how pervasively diabetes casts its net. Maybe then, she believes, more support and understanding would be reached.

In the midst of being a diabetes advocate, training for races and spending time with her husband and their dogs, Rose is busy with her career as a community planner, working with a non-profit community development organization, and was elected president of her state professional organization, the Indiana Chapter of the American Planning Association where she has served on the board for more than a decade. Yet, she always makes time to serve as a Lay Eucharistic Minister for her church.

We salute Rose Scovel, Type 2 advocate and—yes—diabetic athlete—for her inspiring accomplishments, buoyant enthusiasm and steadfast determination to a healthy lifestyle despite diabetes. The Sisterhood of Diabetes supports and thanks Rose with great gusto and encouragement.   ❧

EMILY CHEUNG

Harvard, Yale and a Paris Marathon

Electricity was in the air. The Paris Marathon started and ended at the Arc de Triomphe, and bands were set up to play every two kilometers. The route went along the Seine River, past the Eiffel Tower, while people cheered all along the way.

Emily had trained for one year and her goal was to run the race in under five hours. She used a program of running for seven minutes and walking one minute. She was equipped with a Velcro belt which carried her pump, glucose meter, candy and "Gu" gel packets (a gel sugar + potassium combination often used by athletes for quick energy). Water stops provided orange slices and bananas which helped fill in for nourishment. For the last two miles she sprinted to cross the finish line. She crossed at 4:38:41! It was her most heartfelt success and she glowed with pride to have accomplished this 26.2 mile run. *Ooh-la-la* Emily!

Emily grew up as a happy and healthy youth in Boston, Massachusetts. Diagnosed with diabetes at age thirteen, she still achieved excellent grades throughout school and played on the high school field hockey team.

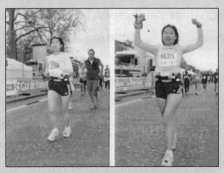

Emily Cheung, Paris marathon

In fact, one summer she worked at Boston's Clara Barton Diabetes Camp for girls as a counselor and field hockey instructor. Besides this, Emily was part of a volunteer group that helped run weekly senior citizen dinner programs at Boston's Lahey Clinic where she played piano and researched songs from the 1930s and '40s that the seniors would recognize from their youth.

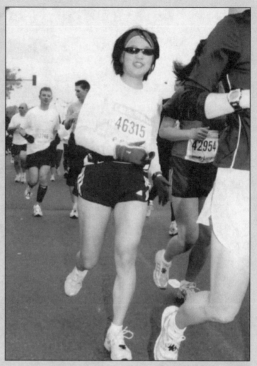

Emily, still smiling

During her under-graduate years at Harvard where she earned a Bachelor's degree in history of science, with a concentration on the history of Chinese and American medicine and behavioral biology, Emily was on the board of a student volunteer group called MIHNUET (Music in Hospitals and Nursing Homes Using Entertainment as Therapy). They connected student musicians with local hospitals and nursing homes to play music for patients and their families. The love and appreciation of music is something that runs deep in Emily's spirit.

Music and running helped keep her diabetes in balance while she earned a Master's degree in public health at Yale. Currently she works with physicians and administrators at a large California healthcare organization to improve quality of care.

Thank you, Emily Cheung, for your music and your commitment to others, reminding us that life is good and life with diabetes is good—even if complicated sometimes. ჯჯ

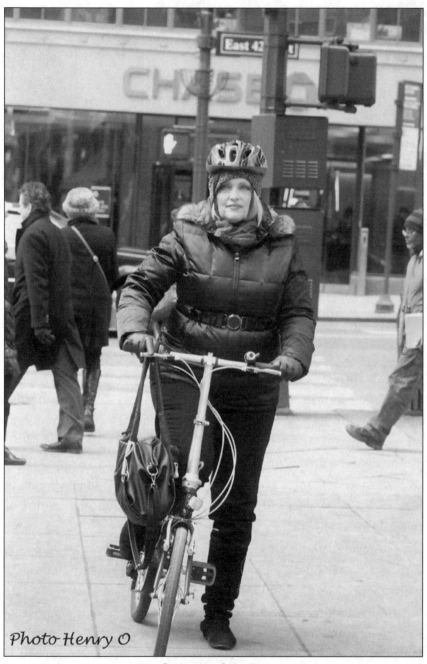

Photo Henry O

Catherine Schuller

Divabetic Pre-Diabetic Biker

What is a Divabetic? Max Szadek, founder and CEO of Divabetic, defines it as a lifestyle that encourages every woman affected by diabetes to take on a bold, sassy personae and posture to help improve the quality of her life. The philosophy of Divabetic, "Glam more—Fear less," empowers women with diabetes. Catherine Schuller lives up to the Divabetic image as a sterling example of a woman with a fulfilling life who also keeps her pre-diabetes at bay so it does not develop into Type 2 diabetes. As Catherine's good friend, Mother Love of Divabetic, reminds her sister divas: "If I have diabetes, I may as well make it look good." And Catherine excels at doing just that.

At age fifty-three, during a routine doctor's visit, Catherine received some shocking news. She was told that she was a prime candidate for insulin resistance, and that "deeper" blood work would be needed to help make a determination. Her doctor's concern was due to the skin tags on her neck (little warts that appear enigmatically in clusters on the surface of the skin) and because of her difficulty losing weight.

The detailed blood tests came back positive for pre-diabetes. Once she recovered from the initial surprise of the diagnosis, Catherine understood why she had been experiencing ongoing weight management problems. A calorie was not a calorie in her case. It was insulin resistance or pre-diabetes causing both the nagging weight situation and recurring skin tags.

Before Pre-Diabetes

Catherine Schuller had left her hometown of Pittsburgh at age twenty-one to pursue a dream of becoming an actress and model in New York City. She had always been creative and aspired to a career in the arts. One of the demands in the industry was an obsession with "thinness."

Catherine was never able to get her weight down below 160 pounds, the weight she settled into after college. At five foot ten, 160 pounds wouldn't have been considered "fat" in the real world. But agents and casting directors tortured her to slim down to 120 pounds.

Pre-Diabetes

Diabetes Mellitus has become a catch-all name for a group of metabolic diseases and conditions characterized by hyperglycemia and impaired production of insulin in the pancreas. Pre-diabetes is often described as that grey area of diabetes where some but not all diagnostic criteria for diabetes are present. The standards set by the American Diabetes Association to determine pre-diabetes are: fasting blood glucose level of 100-125 and Hemoglobin A1C blood test of 5.7-6.4.

The American College of Endocrinology (ACE) and the American Association of Clinical Endocrinologists (AACE) offer lifestyle prevention guidelines for pre-diabetes. By following these strategies, a further diagnosis of Type 2 diabetes may be prevented.

1. Healthy meals—which means following a low fat, low sugar (including simple carbohydrates) and low salt diet.
2. Physical activity—the suggestion is for forty-five minutes of moderate aerobic exercise five days a week. This could be as simple as walking, bicycling or dancing to your favorite music.
3. Reducing weight by as little as five to ten percent can have a significant impact on overall health and well being.

She struggled daily with slimming down her statuesque frame, but to no avail. Catherine was also afraid of a recurrence of the bulimia she battled with in high school. The bulimia came from a motivation to starve herself in order to look like Twiggy, a wildly popular fashion model of the '70s era who was rail thin. Besides starving herself and resorting to bulimic practices whenever she overate, Catherine walked—two miles to and from school each day. But at five foot ten and 133 pounds, she still felt huge.

The plus-size modeling field did not exist in those days and she was left to conform to the standards of the "normal" world. Shortly after her arrival In New York, in between the hustle and bustle of running from audition to audition, an acting teacher encouraged Catherine to take dance classes in order to enhance her presence as an actress.

She signed up for tap and jazz, danced every day, and loved it. Although she was quite lithe and limber, she had quite a bit of catching up to do to keep the pace with the other dancers who had started dance and ballet when they were much younger.

Catherine studied dance for over ten years. She also joined a gym and got a personal trainer to help with strength training to burn off more calories and get in some extra cardio work, even though New York is a cardio city. People walk all over town in addition to sprinting up and down subway steps.

One day her trainer suggested she try cycling around the city in between dance classes and gym visits, and this came as a bright flash of discovery for Catherine. She loved cycling. She had found her sport.

Living in a city like New York, traveling by bicycle has many advantages. It saves on taxi fares, is good for the environment, burns about 300-400 extra calories a day, tones and strengthens glut and thigh muscles and, in Catherine's case, was a fun and wacky way to ride around the city ... dressed in heels and flowing scarves, flashing a smile of confidence. She even bought a sign for her basket that said, "Don't Ask. I'm Saving Gas." But still, every time she stopped to wait for a red light, people would ask why she rode a bike around town. She also joined a group called "Transportation Alternative" in which she met other New Yorkers who opted for the "one less car" mentality.

Catherine has been known to breeze through forty miles in a day on her trusty bike. After having thirty-five bikes stolen over the years in the city, she learned about foldable bikes. These days she rides a Dahon. This foldable bike weighs about thirty pounds, making for some good upper body strengthening as well as cardio work. On rainy or snowy days she heads for the gym and a spin class to keep her wheels in motion.

Catherine went the route of acting and modeling by way of standup comedy. She created a comedy group called "The Nerve." During one of her comedy cabaret shows an agent from Ford Models asked if she would like to join the newly emerging plus-size model group. This was a new concept to Catherine. Suddenly she was the right size and found her niche. She worked in this field for twenty-five years and was recently awarded the Icon of the Industry Award for her contribution to the plus-size modeling world.

Acting, dancing, cycling, playing classical violin with a symphony orchestra—The Symphony Chorus—and Ma Kirtan, a musical group that does *bhakti* (devotional) chanting for the yoga community, kept her life a whirlwind of motion. But then Catherine decided to study design at Parsons School of Design, and from there she created an image-consulting business for full-figured customers called "Curve Style–Reshaping Fashion."

Managing a Pre-Diabetes Lifestyle

When Catherine was diagnosed with the condition of pre-diabetes in July 2007, it was important that she make some adjustments in food choices. The biggest change was to eliminate simple carbohydrates such as sugar, white bread and even pasta, rice and potatoes from her diet. She found an endocrinologist, Dr. Noel Maclaren, to work with whose advice she trusted, and so Catherine lost forty-three pounds and felt great. Her numbers lined up like magic too, with her triglycerides going from 330 to 64 in three short months.

But Then ...

In 2007 Catherine suffered a stroke and was rushed to the hospital. The stroke, not pre-diabetes related, caused paralysis on her right side. It was caused by a congenital condition called PFO (holes in the heart), which she had had since birth. While in the hospital, DNA testing determined that she also had a genetic clotting gene factor, which had probably caused her to develop a clot in her leg (which then traveled through the two holes in her heart and up to the brain, taking out her mobility on the right side).

Catherine underwent surgery to repair the holes in her heart and learned to walk again. She recovered almost fully after hospital treatment and rehab, and after only a month, our gal was back on her bike as though nothing had ever happened. Having a stroke can cause complications if the body is ravaged by the trials and tribulations of poor self-care. But, harnessing her pre-diabetes as well as she does was the key factor to Catherine's rapid and successful recovery. As she proudly notes: "I think it was so great that I had lost forty-three pounds. When I had to get back on my feet (and bike) it was so much easier not having the added burden of extra pounds."

Diabetes Positive

Having diabetes has changed Catherine's life in positive ways that she is grateful for. Insulin resistance is something that *can be controlled and prevented* from growing into Type 2 diabetes. The healthy lifestyle she adopted, and truly enjoys, has also provided Catherine with a powerful platform from which to educate other plus-size women about the dangers of obesity. She counsels that by losing just twenty percent of total body weight and exercising thirty minutes a day a person can impact their diabetes control by fifty-eight percent, leading to good glucose control, lower blood pressure, stress management and many other health benefits.

Catherine has become a much loved volunteer with the Divabetic group. She offers lifestyle and fashion advice, as well as providing inspiration to other women who live with diabetes, paving the way to encourage them all to be "divas." As she says:

> *I think more and more people are finding ways to grab their personal brass rings and run with what they have been dealt, without being angry and resentful. They find ways to slowly tweak and make changes they can live with on a day-to-day basis. They seek out support groups, advice and counseling, meditation and affirmations. In other words, they go for the gold in their lives.*

By incorporating all the positive strides she has made in her life into habits, a healthy lifestyle has become second nature for Catherine. These are choices she *wants* to make rather than *needs* to or *has* to make. Catherine believes it is time we all say NO, in a clear and firm voice, to the packaged and processed foods and the sedentary lifestyle that is gradually consuming and tearing away at people's health. She presents the case for living a consciously healthy life with pre-diabetes as "keeping it at bay like a bomb that never goes off so damage is never done." That's the best she can hope for and work toward.

Catherine's manifesto is:

> *To decree that we have the right to be free of toxic imposed living. If freedom still matters, we can start by living our lives as examples of this—right here—right now. This is what diabetes has taught me. I was asleep about my health, now I am awake and sharing this message with others. If truth be told, this is the hopeful message I wish to inspire about living with diabetes. It is a message you can wear in your mind and heart 24/7.*

We all have the means to harness our own good health. Catherine's message and manifesto is one everybody reading this book can and should embrace. As part of the Sisterhood of Diabetes we support Catherine's message and resolve to make our diabetes look good, as is the philosophy of Divabetic.

Thanks, Catherine Schuller, for brightening our smiles. ❦

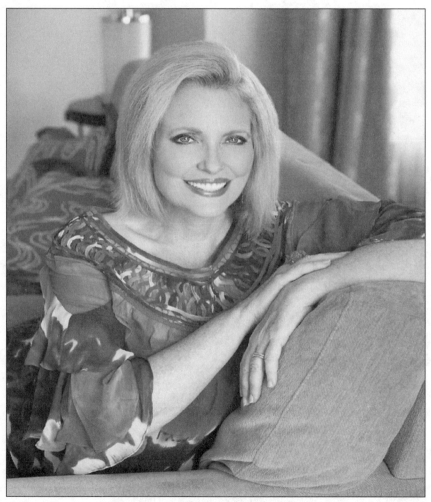

Catherine, spokeswoman for good health

CHAPTER 7

Surmounting the Insurmountable

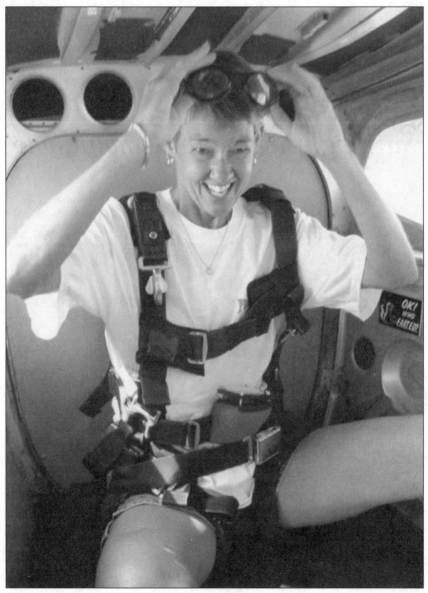

Suzi Vietti

Flying Low and Slow

S uzi Vietti believes that knowledge is the precious key that unlocks doors and motivates us to succeed. She uses herself as the perfect example. It took Suzi many long years, tough times and multiple challenges to apply her "key theory" and accomplish her dream of becoming a successful athlete. When she gives talks to children and teens with diabetes, her hope is that they look at her and say, "Wow! This lady has really done a lot in her life even though she has lived with diabetes for nearly fifty years!" When this book went to press, Suzi was sixty-four years old and still moving.

If Suzi Vietti was around during the Renaissance period of history, more than likely she would have been pals with Leonardo DaVinci. Instead, Suzi is a modern day Renaissance gal. She paints, decorates, teaches, lectures, pilots an airplane, climbs rocks and runs half-marathons. Navigating the maze of such accomplishments, Suzi, besides living with Type 1 diabetes, has had some serious breaks, bruises and illnesses in her lifetime.

The Beginning

Suzi began her life with diabetes at age fourteen in the southeast corner of Kansas, in a small town called Girard. Her father had been a stellar soldier in World War II, as a forward observer on the German front lines. His position was both stressful and dangerous. Not only was her father the only one in his battalion to make it home alive, but he holds the distinction of being the most decorated soldier from Kansas. Tragically, after the war his life changed. He started to drink, and eventually the alcoholism took over and had a disastrous effect on his wife and young daughter Suzi.

When her father was having a really bad night, Suzi and her mom would head into town for an ice cream cone, a coke and some candy bars to escape the unhappiness and lack of communication at home. Once Suzi was diagnosed with diabetes, she and her mom still went into town but sipped on diet cokes, skipped the candy bars and now and then indulged in an ice cream cone. During those troubled years, she became her mother's caretaker and the two held onto the close bond they built with each other in hard times until her mother's death in 2000.

Back in the 1950s, diabetes education was limited to a week's tour of duty in the hospital—this included injecting an orange with saline solution to learn the technique of giving insulin injections, and practicing the art of urine testing using an eye dropper and test tube. Scare tactics were also applied about kidney, eye, heart and circulatory problems that could occur and wounds that would not heal. "I also learned at age fourteen that child-bearing was very difficult for diabetics," Suzi recalls. She also remembers leaving the hospital as an impressionable young teenager armed with many fears and a determination not to be "different" from anyone else.

Because of all the sadness and upheaval Suzi experienced as a child and teenager, in later years she and her husband Bill devoted themselves to raising their own family with the comfort of love and communication. They celebrate close family ties and respect for one another, as well as a determination never to hide family problems. If something arises, they deal with it head on.

Shaping the Athlete

Many happy memories from Suzi's youth helped balance the sad ones. She fondly recalls water-skiing with her three cousins on the nearby lake, every day, from the time school ended in June until it re-opened in September. She loved water skiing, in addition to competing with her cousins. During the other seasons, she was devoted to both riding and training horses. She loved competing with friends and relatives, and did so, setting extremely high standards for herself. But when it came time to compete in school or team sports, her motivation and interest dwindled. Perhaps it was because, at that time, choices for girls were limited to softball and track.

Trying To Fit In

Being different from the other kids at school became obvious to Suzi, especially since food was involved in just about every activity she and her friends did, especially in high school and later during college years. Few sugar-free options were available, and at that time sugar of any sort was a strict no-no for diabetes. Balancing carbohydrates and exercise, fast acting insulin and carb counting were not on the horizon yet. The rule was simple—no sugar permitted. When all her friends ordered Cokes, Suzi was stuck with plain water, or non-sweetened limeade, or nothing, which she felt made her stand out from the crowd. It was even worse when they went out after games for burgers or pizza. Being the odd one, as a teenager, was not something anyone aspired to in the 1960s in Kansas.

At that time, the recommended insulin regimen was one shot of NPH insulin a day. In order to keep blood glucose balanced with this type of treatment, it was necessary to follow a very tight time line with meals and insulin peaks; not an easy task for anyone, especially a self-conscious teenager with Type 1 diabetes. In college, where drinking alcohol was commonplace, Suzi got herself into some dangerous situations while trying to negotiate beer with insulin action.

Adulthood

Fortunately, life changed after college. Suzi had met the love of her life, Bill Vietti, in high school. In 1972 they married. In 1976 she gave birth to a ten-pound-twelve-ounce son. Two years later, another son was born, but sadly he only survived four days due to medical complications. Suzi remembers people asking if the reason for the baby's death was due to her diabetes. The question played on her and became destructive to her mental stability. She took on full responsibility for her son's death even though she understood the reality that other circumstances were at play besides her diabetes. Although her doctor told her she should not attempt to have more children, Suzi and Bill became resolute about trying again. One year later her doctor felt she could try for one more pregnancy. The outcome was beautiful twin daughters. Life was wonderful again.

Off Balance

By 1987 Suzi began focusing on blood sugars, weight and insulin quantities to an unhealthy extreme. Thinking that she must achieve the perfect balance at all times, weight gain became an obsessive fear, and her excessive measures led to bulimia and depression. Suzi dealt with high blood sugars by exercising way beyond her limits of being insulin dependent. Overeating followed by abusing diuretics for fear of gaining weight established a dangerous pattern.

Finally, in trying to step outside herself and view her actions more objectively to conquer these problems, Suzi discovered that such behavior was not uncommon for people with diabetes. Using her powers of inner strength, coupled with some good therapy and three hospitalizations, Suzi recuperated to a healthy lifestyle. Hers was a difficult road to travel and she worries about others with diabetes experiencing the same difficulties. To help prevent this problem, Suzi speaks to local diabetes groups regarding diabetes and eating disorders.

New Adventures

In the early 1990s, Suzi began running. She loved the feeling of being able to run distances she never thought she could. Over time, and with plenty of low blood sugar corrections, she managed to get the running and diabetes to become friends. More understanding and better education helped explain how to balance insulin, blood sugars and extended exercise, as Suzi built up her distance running gradually and with great pride.

In 2002, at age fifty-two, Suzi became interested in piloting her husband's

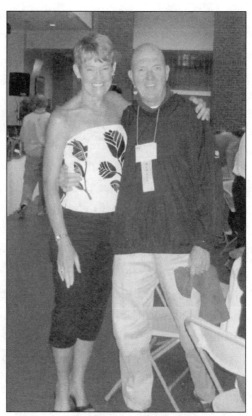

Suzi and Bill, Boston DESA banquet

powered parachute plane. That same year she tested for and became licensed as a Basic Flight Instructor, and also took her first tandem sky dive. Thrilling!

A Frightening Diagnosis

When Suzi and Bill drove to Colorado to visit their three grown children in 2003, she noticed some numbness in the bottoms of both feet. The previous day she had run five miles and felt just fine. But now the numbness increased until she could barely walk. By the time she was admitted to the emergency room in a hospital in Colorado Springs, the numbness had reached her waist. The immediate fear was that it would travel to her diaphragm and compromise her ability to breathe.

After what seemed like an artillery barrage of tests, a diagnosis of Transverse Myelitis was confirmed. Transverse Myelitis is a rare autoimmune disease that affects one to four people in a million. The immune system aggressively attacks the spinal cord mistaking it for a foreign substance. There is no cure, but steroids are often administered intravenously to repair the immune system. In Suzi's case, the combination of steroids and diabetes was like fire and ice, and her blood sugar peaked out at eight hundred before getting back under control. Decidedly she was frightened, and wondered what fate had in store for her with this condition. For their part, the doctors nodded in agreement that she would never run, fly or drive again. There was a possibility that she might not even walk. But for Suzi, this news was the defining moment. She decided with bullish determination that she would prove them wrong.

While it took some time before she could stand up without falling over, as soon as she could manage that she started an aggressive program of physical therapy. After many frustrating months, she regained her balance and finally began to walk again. Eventually, she even started a movement that might best be described as a "wobbling run."

As her strength returned, Suzi prepared herself for the next challenge—in the form of a bicycle. Although biking was a painful task, she stuck with it and eventually got to the point of really enjoying it. By then she had clearly determined not to sit and watch her world go by from a wheelchair or a bed. She would run, bike, drive, climb, hike and fly through life.

At this critical time, her daughters challenged Suzi to run a half-marathon with them, and she took on that challenge. Ten short months later they completed the Boulder Backroads Run, her first half-marathon, which coincided, incidentally, with the fortieth anniversary of her diabetes diagnosis. Suzi was running again (not looking back), and driving—solo, in fact, from Kansas to Colorado to run the race. Shortly after that success, she began working towards achieving her next goal—to get back in the seat of her plane.

Seeing how well Suzi was leaping over every obstacle that crossed her path, Bill encouraged his wife to put on her pilot's cap and fly her powered parachute again. By now the PPC Ultra lights were under the domain of the Federal Aviation Administration., and a new license and classification was created called "Sport Pilot." The test was a rigorous oral, written and practical one, but the result was extraordinary. In May 2005, Suzi Vietti became the first woman Sport Pilot in America. Soon after that Suzi and Bill created the group called "PPC Caravans" and set up their own website for it (*www.ppcpilot.com*). Within a short time they were flying their parachutes with friends while on vacation. Thus far, in 2014, they have flown in all forty-eight lower states and seen some of the most beautiful parts of America from the air. They also have a new plane. Their goal is still to fly all fifty! "Flying," as Suzi says, "low and slow."

The moment you take off you leave all your worries and cares on the ground. From up above, you see all God's creations of wildlife and beautiful terrain. Sometimes there is no other spot in the country that has a similar topographical layout as the one you see at a given moment from the air. There is nothing comparable.

Rock Climbing, Too

In the life of someone such as Suzi Vietti, a new discovery is always waiting in the wings. She found one in the sport and challenge of rock climbing. As her daughters live in Colorado, the Rocky Mountain state, what better place was there to climb rocks?

First attempts were somewhat tenuous. Suzi felt a bit unsure of her legs and sense of balance, but after a few tries the rocks became her friends and offered her another sport to enjoy. Suzi also had a close

What Is a Powered Parachute?

The Powered Parachute is a simple airframe with seats for a pilot and passenger, and is the safest and most economical way to experience sport aviation today. They fly at a safe and constant 28 mph, are resistant to stalls, and you can't loop it or dive it. The Powered Parachute is the best way to experience the world from a low, slow and safe perspective.

How Does It Work?

The canopy is positioned on the ground behind the aircraft for takeoff. As the pilot adds power and the aircraft begins to roll forward, the canopy inflates and rotates overhead. After carefully checking the inflated canopy, the pilot adds full power to climb out. The Powered Parachute has only two controls, the steering bars and the throttle. Add power and you gain altitude and reduce power to lose altitude. Exerting pressure on the left steering bar results in a left turn and exerting pressure on the right steering bar allows the machine to turn right. Landing is easily mastered. Simply reduce power and line the aircraft up into the wind. As you approach touchdown, pushing forward on both steering bars results in a flare that insures a smooth landing. In the unlikely case that your engine quits, your canopy remains fully inflated and you are able to float back to earth in full control. Setting up to fly at a field takes about fifteen minutes and the aircraft stores easily in a small garage. (This Information comes from Six Chuter Inc. Powered Parachutes, *www.sixchuterchutes.com*)

friend in Arizona who was an expert climber and teacher, and together they climbed Pinnacle Peak in 2007. This extreme accomplishment helped reassure Suzi that she was well on the road to full recovery from the Transverse Myelitis condition.

The Renaissance Woman Re-Emerges

At the beginning of this Renaissance woman's story, it was mentioned that Suzi is an artist. She enjoys working in the faux painting medium. There was a time after the Transverse Myelitis diagnosis when she was quite concerned about her ability, or rather inability, to climb high ladders and scaffolding, let alone paint once she got up there. Like everything else in Suzi's life, however, she focused and conquered the dragon. Today she continues to paint beautiful decorative art on walls and ceilings all over Kansas.

Suzi's life is busy and fruitful. She feels that, in a way, having diabetes helps her get things done ... although life would probably be much easier without it ... as the daily discipline involved in managing diabetes requires timing and organization.

Suzi wants to let people know that they can do many things and accomplish their goals even though they have diabetes; that having diabetes is "not the end of the world." Being prepared and educated about diabetes helps her live "in peace with it," and she hopes that others with diabetes will look at her life as an awakening for themselves.

Surely we, in the Sisterhood of Diabetes, are kindled and fired up with the story of Kansas' own Suzi Vietti.   ⬙⬗

BLAIR RYAN

Give It a Shot

Through all the intricacies of competitive sports, fine tuning diabetes plays a major role. For Blair Ryan, an Ironman athlete with diabetes, the capstone project required for her Master's program was the creation of *www.Giveitashotfilms.com*—a professional multimedia collection that follows ten athletes with diabetes training for an Ironman triathlon.

Blair also completed a 10,982-mile drive of the nation in her Toyota Matrix to visit the homes each of the 2010-2011 Captains of Triabetes (a factor of Insulindependence) while they trained for an Ironman race that, at the time of the visits, was ten months out. Insulindependence also sent Blair on assignment to Hawaii for the final Captain's visit. While there, Blair documented the experiences of a new Triabetes club member competing in her first full Ironman, the Ford Ironman World Championship, despite having been diagnosed with Type 1 diabetes eight weeks before the event.

The athletes of Insulindependence are showing the world the stamina, talent, dedication, courage and goals a person with diabetes can realize. The diabetes community has produced Olympic gold medalists, sub-nine hour Ironman athletes and successful summits of Mt. Everest.

While the crucial importance of exercise in controlling diabetes cannot be emphasized enough, still many newly diagnosed patients are discouraged from continuing activities they have done throughout their lives or are precluded from taking on physical challenges. You will enjoy the outstanding creative work Blair is doing to counter this misunderstanding through her films. *Give It a Shot* shows her passion for sending this message, loud and clear. This change in philosophy from hiding diabetes to promoting it through her work came when Blair realized that not everyone had the support she did. As she witnessed this, she developed the desire to protect those newly diagnosed with Type 1 diabetes from misconceptions about life with diabetes.

In a sense Blair has turned diabetes into an art form through her videos and films.

She wants to be a photojournalist and travel the world in hopes of changing it for the better through her work. For now she is doing just that, but close to home in California, where she has taken the position of Media and Publications Director for Insulin-

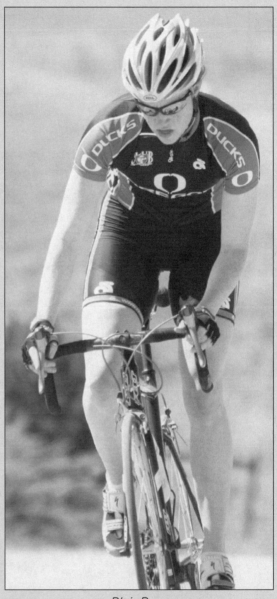

Blair Ryan

dependence. We wish Blair Ryan, athlete and artist, our support as we stand together as pillars of inspiration in the Sisterhood of Diabetes.   ✤

CHAPTER 8

Moving With Body, Mind and Diabetes

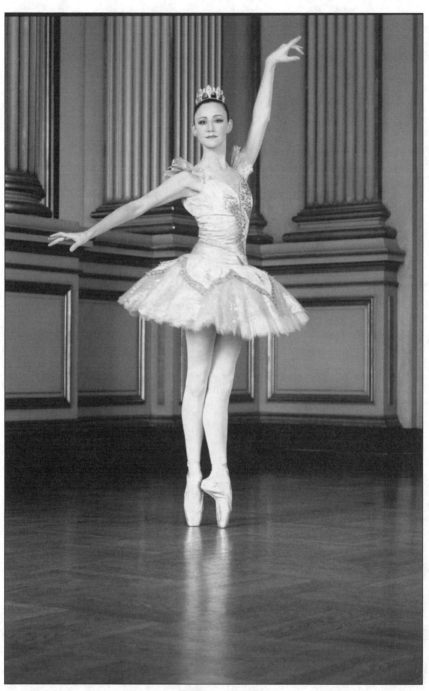

Zippora Karz

ZIPPORA KARZ

The Leap Within the Dancer

Many of us reach for the coffee pot for our morning "wake-up." A dancer stretches and lengthens, points and flexes, for an hour and a half before beginning the rigors of a six-hour rehearsal day. When evening comes, it's makeup, costumes and a performance. This is the life of a soloist ballerina.

Yes, dance is unquestionably athletic.

In 1971, at age six, Zippora Karz took her first dance class in Bangkok, Thailand. Zippora's father, a cardiologist, had volunteered to go there during the Vietnam War. While in Bangkok, Zippora, her older sister Michele and their mother took Thai dance lessons. The beauty and grace of the movements provided her first insight into the transformative power of dance. She also loved the long, curved, brass fingernails their teacher wore, and she too longed to wear nails like that to dance in class. Her mother explained that she was too young to wear brass fingernails in class, but she bought them for Zippora and her sister to wear during their home talent shows and on special occasions. Zippora loved the feeling of doing the precision hand and head movements as much as she loved wearing beautiful, Thai silk robes ... and of course her brass nails.

A year later, back home in California, their mother asked Zippora and Michele if they wanted to take ballet lessons. Michele said yes, and so Zippora said yes as well. At first Zippora didn't really like ballet and wanted to quit. She was bored with trying to put her body in positions with toes pointed out to the sides; it felt strained and unnatural to her. She preferred horseback riding or playing with her dogs and cats. However, most days, as she waited to be picked up after dance class, Zippora peeked to watch the advanced class dance and leap. There was such vibrant energy in that room that she fantasized what it would be like to dance with such freedom and power. The next year she would qualify for that class, Sheila's class. So she decided not to quit.

Falling in Love

In her third year of ballet school in Sheila's class, Zippora fell in love and became impassioned with dance. The more her body became a refined instrument, the more she felt transported by the music. Her perceptive teacher recognized Zippora's gift and encouraged her to audition for the summer program at the world renowned School of American Ballet, the official school of the New York City Ballet. She was accepted!

After Zippora's second summer at SAB, she was asked to stay on as a full-time winter student. Sheila immediately spoke with Zippora's mother about the importance of this opportunity. Up to this point, although Zippora loved to dance, she had not really dreamt about becoming a ballerina. And so, without knowing much about what lay ahead, and with her mother's blessing, the fifteen-year-old dancer moved to New York City and a life of hard work, rigorous discipline, sweat, sore feet, and flashes of magic, great joy and the passion of dance. Zippora soon found herself surrounded by the legends of the dance world from George Balanchine to Jerome Robbins to Nureyev, Baryshnikov, Peter Martins, Suzanne Farrell and all the great dancers of the New York City Ballet. A world she had never known opened to her and her heart began to dream of a life on the stage.

The Gene Pool

That essence, that leap within the dancer, was in Zippora's gene pool. Her grandmother Gloria performed a solo act in vaudeville and danced throughout her life. Her mother Ellen had studied modern dance at Juilliard and continued to dance traditional folk dances throughout her life. Zippora and her sisters often accompanied their mother to folk dance camps where they would all dance together. On occasion, their grandmother would choreograph a piece for all three generations to dance together. Though her mother began performing at a young age and trained at Juilliard, she started her formal training too late to pursue a professional career. Should her three daughters, Michele, Zippora and Romy ever desire to dance, Ellen wanted her girls to have the opportunity to experience the artistic as well as the technical brilliance of ballet. And so, when they returned from Thailand, and when Ellen heard about Sheila, the exceptional ballet teacher who ran a studio near their home in Los Angeles, she suggested that the girls begin to study there.

By the age of eighteen, Zippora was a full member of the prestigious N.Y. company and at twenty-seven she had worked her way to reach the

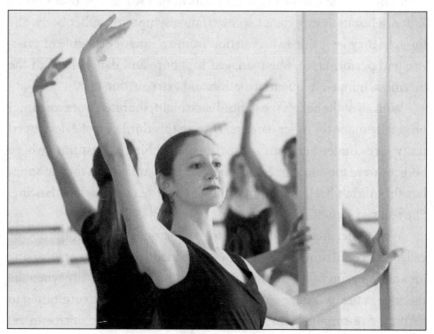

Zippora: model of art and grace

dream of every ballerina, that of becoming a soloist. This position came with the creative and artistic opportunity to dance the ballets of George Balanchine and Jerome Robbins of the New York City Ballet. Zippora danced the part of the Sugarplum Fairy in "The Nutcracker," a Muse in Balanchine's "Apollo," and other select roles. Although the rigors of professional dance are strict and without mercy, Zippora loved the days of leaping and turning, jumping and moving and feeling at one with the music. Her body responded. These moments were so magical and uplifting that she worked even harder to discover how much more she could achieve.

Enter Diabetes

With her history of hard work, discipline, self motivation and love of artistic expression, the world of dance became a natural habitat to find joy, happiness, creativity and magic in her life. But, in her third year, towards the end of the winter season of 1987, at age twenty-one, Zippora began to experience some strange symptoms in her body. She thought they were due to exhaustion from an intense schedule of practice and performance. She managed to ignore and dance through the dizziness, hunger, frequent urination and extreme thirst.

With all of the ballets she danced each night, she often wore costumes originally made for other dancers. During this third year she developed nasty sores under her arms caused by the rubbing of costumes whose bodices were too long for her frame. She took antibiotics for the sores, but they didn't heal, making it difficult to lift her arms while dancing. She realized something was wrong.

With reluctance, Zippora went to the doctor. A week later the doctor called … several times, but Zippora was so maddeningly busy rehearsing for an important role that she put off retuning the call. Finally, when the message at the backstage entrance read "Urgent," Zippora committed to taking a five-minute break between rehearsals to call the doctor to get her lab results.

Responding to the demand to come into the office right away, Zippora was told that the lab results confirmed diabetes; was advised that they needed to discuss a treatment plan, at another time, and was handed some pamphlets warning of the complications of uncontrolled diabetes—heart disease, stroke, kidney failure, blindness and loss of limbs being some of the highlights.

Zippora listened to these dire warnings for a few minutes, then zipped back to the theater just in time to put on thick false eye lashes, draw long extended black lines under and around her eyes, outline and then color in her lips, and get into costume. This was her nightly routine for entering her world of magic and beauty that is ballet. She performed that night.

Diabetes Denial

Zippora was healthy, active, and successful, and was now being told that her life would change now and forever. No wonder her initial response was complete denial. She knew diabetes as a disease that people donated money to at charity events at the ballet, but she refused to believe that diabetes could possibly have anything to do with *her*.

Zippora tried to convince herself that the numbers would go back to normal once she got some much needed rest … or else … or else … that it had simply been a lab error. What made it even more confusing for her was that she was put on oral medication. The doctor's diagnosis clearly assumed she had Type 2 diabetes.

As we have noted in other cases of the amazing Sisterhood of Diabetes, Zippora's lifestyle of exercise, healthy eating habits, discipline and positive attitude made her a natural candidate for optimal diabetes management. She was headstrong, a hard worker, and capable of putting her nose to the grindstone and studying, studying and studying more So when she heard the Type 2 diagnosis, she felt relieved in a sense to know that her healthy eating habits and constant exercise could potentially reverse this diabetes "annoyance." Her strategy worked well—for a while.

Zippora was in a "honeymoon phase" of diabetes that sometimes occurs for a brief period post-diagnosis, when a small amount of insulin is still being produced. Once the honeymoon was over, however, a new diagnosis of Type 1 (Insulin Dependent Diabetes Mellitus) was given. Now there could be no denial—no amount of exercise or perfect diet would create the insulin that Zippora needed to carry on her life as a ballerina.

Questioning the Ability to Cope

Reacting to the daunting reality of administering insulin while exercising up to twelve hours a day, Zippora felt her world had come crashing down. As she learned how to juggle insulin shots with her intense performance schedule, she actually started to question whether ballet was a realistic lifestyle for an insulin dependent diabetic. A dancer needs to feel every part of her body from her fingertips to her toes, not to mention giving the pinpoint focus required for a great performance. When her sugars were the slightest bit off kilter, she lost that vital connection and concentration. Plus, with the amount of exercise required throughout the day, she felt like she was constantly on the verge of going hypoglycemic.

It took years of struggling and strategizing until Zippora learned how to dance successfully with diabetes, and mainly through trial and error, since there were no role models or reference points she could use for comparison or guidance. Some important lessons she garnered along this winding and sometimes jagged path were:

- Never take a shot of insulin right before a performance (unless blood sugar is way too high). The exercise will lower blood sugar levels and continue to do so post exercising.
- If blood sugars are indeed a bit higher during the show, learn to accept that the performance might not be as perfect as desired. Let go of trying to be perfect to fulfill personal potential every

performance. Accept a new potential as a person with diabetes, one that puts personal health and well being first.

- Always carry nuts and seeds and dried fruit in a dance bag and keep it close to the wing of the stage in case a quick snack is needed.
- Between scenes, if feeling a low blood sugar, have a strategy in place the works well. Chewing on a couple of dates will raise blood glucose quickly, thereby allowing entering the stage with a good blood sugar.
- During the day keep toes clean and dry. Wear white cotton socks. Soak feet in Epsom Salts and use DEI or Tinactin powder at first sign of a toe blister or corn.

Like all the other Sisters in this book, Zippora rose to the challenge. At the time of her diagnosis she felt that having to take shots of insulin indicated that her body was failing. Eventually she came to accept and feel grateful for insulin. She understood that it was allowing her to continue to live her passion.

Zippora continued to dance with the New York City Ballet for thirteen years after her diagnosis, sixteen years in total. Seven of these years she danced brilliantly as a soloist ballerina. Dancing Balanchine ballets night after night was an honor she never took for granted.

Time to Leap onto Other Stages

After sixteen years as a professional ballerina, Zippora Karz passed her tutus and tiaras and toe shoes on to the next generation of ballerinas and retired from her position with the New York City Ballet. She began to stage performances as répétiteur (instructor and supervisor) for the Balanchine Trust, working with dance companies, universities, and schools throughout the U.S. and Europe, teaching the masterpieces she had been honored to dance. She continues to enjoy this work. Zippora also teaches master dance classes.

Her passionate desire to make the earth a healthier place for all of us to live in has become an avocation. For her, health is physical, emotional, psychological and spiritual as it relates to individuals and the universe, and Zippora believes and lives by the principles of helping people become more aware and connected to their lives and to those around them. While she has experimented with different ways to eat, she has always believed in eating fresh, vibrant, plant-based foods (preferably organic), high-quality protein (no hormones or antibiotics), and healthy fats. Her favorite meal might consist of high-quality organically-raised protein, avocados, nuts and seeds, fresh veggies, leafy greens and plenty of early-harvest olive oil and /or pesto sauce.

I asked Zippora what would be the most important message for her to send out as a role model. She answered: "We must be responsible for our health. We must find a passion, something of meaning that motivates and drives us to take better care of ourselves. We can live full, healthy, passion-filled lives with diabetes."

Zippora devotes much time to speaking at diabetes conferences where she also enjoys teaching movement. I have seen her in action at CWD (Children With Diabetes) conferences as she captures the hearts of the audience of kids. They recognize the common bond of diabetes and they see the magic and sparkle of the Sugarplum Fairy in her.

Zippora has published her memoirs in a book titled *The Sugarless Plum*. You can find it on her website *www.zipporakarz.com*. It is a fascinating and magical read that will surely make you want to dance.

We are so proud and fortunate to have Zippora Karz as a shining star in the Sisterhood of Diabetes. ❧

MELITTA RORTY

Diabetes and Yoga: The Perfect Balance

In 2006, when I was editor of *The DESA Challenge* newsletter for diabetes, sports and exercise, Melitta Rorty sent me an article about her passion for the practice of yoga. Until then most of the articles in the *The Challenge* were stories about mainstream and extreme sports: cycling, running, dog sled racing, swimming, mountaineering and the like. I found Melitta's article on yoga's benefits for diabetes uniquely interesting, and have included it in this chapter, from the Winter 2007 issue, for you to enjoy.

The Corpse Pose (*Savasana*) That Got Her
Melitta was thirty-four years old when she took her first yoga class. At the end of the practice they did a pose called "Savasana," the corpse pose, which consists of breathing with concentration into each part of the body, beginning with the toes, tightening and then a total release, with a deep exhalation. By the time the entire body has been scanned, the student is in a state of profound relaxation. At that moment, Melitta fell passionately in love with the practice of yoga. As she says, "I knew yoga was 'it' for me."

Yoga and Its Benefits for People with Diabetes

By Melitta Rorty

Yoga is an ancient practice that uses poses, breathing techniques, relaxation, and meditation to balance mind, body, and spirit. Yoga originated in India thousands of years ago and takes many forms, but Hatha yoga, which involves stretching the body and forming different poses while keeping breathing slow and controlled, is most commonly practiced in the West. Yoga has much to offer people with diabetes, and probably its greatest benefit is stress reduction. Diabetes is exacerbated by stress, and yoga is a useful tool to reduce stress to both set the stage for overall well-being and to help cope with the tedium associated with our daily diabetes care. High levels of the stress hormones adrenaline and cortisol raise blood glucose levels, thus reducing stress is integral to good blood glucose control. Yoga cannot cure diabetes, but the many benefits of yoga (stress reduction, increased sense of well being, discipline, and focus) can help make daily life with the disease more manageable.

Additionally, yoga can be an important part of a well-rounded fitness program that includes cardiovascular exercise, strengthening, and flex-ibility. Athletes may find the increased flexibility, functional strength, and balance to be an integral part of a holistic fitness regimen. But as described above, the benefits of yoga go far beyond flexibility and functional strength.

Hatha yoga, which incorporates physical poses and breath work, has a number of styles, and it is important to find the style that speaks to you and suits your needs and nature. Hatha yoga styles range from gentle yoga to Iyengar Yoga, which focuses on precision and alignment in poses, to Ashtanga Yoga, which is a strong and vigorous style often favored by athletes. *Yoga Journal* online has a yoga guide that provides summary descriptions of many styles. (www.yogajournal.com/newtoyoga/165_1.cfm).

Timothy McCall, M.D.'s book on yoga and medical conditions, entitled *Yoga as Medicine: The Yogic Prescription for Health and Healing* (Bantam Dell, Summer 2007) contains excellent information on the benefits of stress reduction on diabetes health and yoga contraindications based on the presence of diabetic complications. He talks about yoga as the best stress reduction method ever invented. Yoga has so many tools to offer in its poses, breathing practices, and meditation that there is something for everybody. For people with diabetes, vigorous yoga can cause drops in blood glucose, leading to hypoglycemia. It is important to monitor your blood sugar before and after a yoga session to gauge your reaction to the yoga practice. Typically, yoga practitioners are advised to refrain from eating for several hours before class. Those with diabetes should aim for blood sugar control and not concern themselves with that generic guideline. Anyone with diabetic complications should exercise caution when practicing yoga. People with retinopathy should avoid inversions and any poses that increase pressure in the eyes. Poses such as handstand and downward facing dog should be avoided.

The best way to start a yoga practice is to find a competent teacher with whom you feel comfortable, and whose style suits you. Many yoga studios now offer Yoga Basics classes or an introductory series of yoga classes. These "yoga training wheels" classes can be especially beneficial for those who have no experience with yoga, because even beginning classes can be too advanced for those just starting out.

My personal yoga practice is one year "older" than my type 1 diabetes. Yoga helped me cope in those first confusing months after diagnosis when I believed that diabetes had ruined my life. Yoga and exercise were a refuge. Twelve years have gone by and I am enrolled in a 3-year yoga teacher training/advanced studies program at the Yoga Room in Berkeley, California. I practice yoga these days simply because it makes my life better. I am more fixable physically and I enjoy the mental flexibility my yoga practice provides. ♉

Yoga Resources:
Moving Toward Balance: 8 Weeks of Yoga with Rodney Yee, by Rodney Yee and Nina
    Zolotow (Rodale, 2004).
*Full Catastrophe Living: Using the Wisdom of Your Body and Mind to Face Stress,
    Pain, and Illness.* Jon Kabat-Zinn (Dell Publishing, New York. 1990). (www.
    mindfulnesstapes.com).
Yoga for Beginners II DVD (www.gaiam.com) with Patricia Walden is a very basic
    and accessible beginning yoga practice.

Life Before Yoga

Until that time Melitta had played many different sports. In fact, she discovered her competitive nature when she was seven years old, after coming in third place in a swim meet. That fueled her fire. It was the last time she came in third! She worked with resolve and earnestness for first place from then on.

She recalls that in third grade all the boys wanted to race her in a school running event. She did, and soon breezed past all of them, which made them furious and want to beat her. The teacher had other ideas about this, however. Even though the boys begged the teacher, she would not allow Melitta to race against the boys again. "Whose side was the teacher on?" a female athlete might ask.

By the time Melitta got to Wellesley College she had become a "jock of all sports, master of none." And then she discovered Squash. Her enthusiasm for the game challenged her to try out for the intercollegiate team. She made it! Squash became her sport through her years at school. By graduation, Melitta was honored with both academic recognition and a Scholar-Athlete award.

Through the years she has always been active in the things that make her feel good, healthy and challenged. She has hiked at altitudes of 17,771 feet in the Himalayas, and today a 20-mile hike in the mountains is a like a walk in the park for this enthusiastic, willful athlete. Perhaps this determination is in her genes, since both parents and her two sisters and one brother all enjoy nature, physical activity and sports.

Melitta appreciates her life and her work as a registered professional geologist. Equipped with a BS in geology and an MS in hydrogeology, she works for the Pacific Gas and Electric Company in the San Francisco Bay Area as part of their environmental cleanup group.

Yoga, Diabetes and Competition

One day, about six months after Melitta began studying and practicing yoga—at precisely 3:30 on the afternoon of April 13, 1995 when she was hospitalized in critical condition—she received a diagnosis of Type 2 diabetes. Sadly, it was a blatant misdiagnosis based on age rather than etiology.

Once the correct diagnosis of Type 1 diabetes was confirmed, Melitta pushed herself constantly to prove that she was everything she had been previous to this diagnosis. She ran in 5K races—always finishing within the top three in her age group. She did a mini-triathlon. Over time

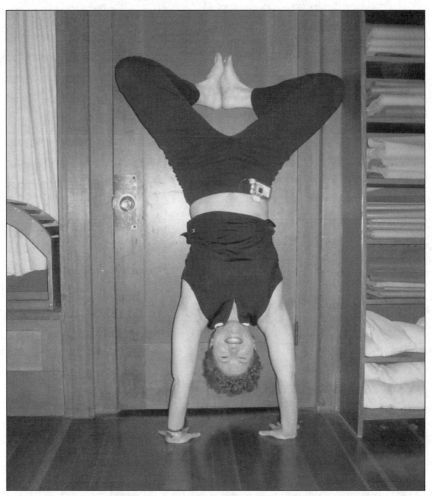

Melitta Rorty . . . handstand with insulin pump!

LATE AUTOIMMUNE DIABETES IN ADULTS

Approximately one percent of the population of athletic and perfectly healthy adults, in the thirty-five-to-forty age range, come down with a condition known as "delayed onset adult juvenile Type 1 diabetes." It is also called LADA, Latent Auto-immune Diabetes in Adults. Some health professionals call it the mysterious "X-factor." It is a slow and gradual onset of Type 1 diabetes in adults that is often mistaken for Type 2 diabetes.

The diagnosis of Type 2 is age based. At the time of diagnosis of Type 2, patients are usually prescribed medications such as Metformin or Sulfonylreas. The drugs may work for an extended period of months or years, until the pancreas stops producing any insulin. Eventually, there is no insulin being produced and the patient's blood glucose levels rise despite prescribed oral meds. The health of the patient can deteriorate to the point of ketoacidosis if proper diagnosis of Type 1 is not discovered and treated accordingly with insulin.

she has come to under-stand diabetes and how to manage it. She has also come to understand that she is, indeed, everything she was before diagnosis.

Life (with Diabetes) Is Worth Living

Melitta doesn't need to prove herself by running races anymore. Now that she has turned fifty, she enjoys pursuing her passion to study yoga at the highest levels. She lives a rewarding life with her partner Brande, and basks in the company of family and many great friends. She also takes time to seek out the best enchiladas in the Bay area (and the best dark chocolate as well) and travel to exotic places whenever the opportunity presents itself. Diabetes has become simply a part of Melitta's life. She uses an insulin pump and Contin-uous Glucose Monitor, and both technologies help with excellent management. Of course there are occasional moments (they can happen to all of us who live with diabetes, no matter how perfectly we try to manage and guide our blood sugars) when she has a bad, low blood sugar. "I hate this *^#*!*!* disease," she shouts out of frustration. But then she balances the numbers and all is well once again. The calm rhythm of yoga and meditation sets in to slow down the diabetes rollercoaster. At the end of the day Melitta believes, "You can live really well with diabetes and you can live your dreams—and kick butt."

Changing Perceptions of Adult Onset Type 1

When Melitta was misdiagnosed with Type 2 diabetes, fifteen years ago, she thought to herself "I bet this is a common occurrence in medicine." She was right. Type 1 diabetes is not exclusively a childhood disease. Over the years she has concentrated her will of steel on changing this misconception. She has written numerous blogs on *www.TuDiabetes. org* about the problem of misdiagnosis. She has approached both the American and Canadian Diabetes Associations about recognizing the prevalence of adult onset Type 1 diabetes and, as a result of her work, information on this topic has been included in Dr. McCall's chapter on diabetes in the authoritative book *Yoga As Medicine: The Yogic Prescription for Health and Healing* (Bantam, 2007).

"I am nowhere near changing the misperception that Type 1 diabetes is a childhood disease," Melitta admits. "I figure that fight is going to take me the rest of my life. My dad lived to be ninety-three and my mom is ninety and doing great. She can hike ten miles. So—I have genetics and time on my side." Meanwhile, Melitta does her best to balance life just like the perfect *Vrksasana* (Standing Like A Tree) pose.

We thank Melitta for her inspiration and enlightenment about yoga practice, which everyone in the Sisterhood of Diabetes can incorporate into her exercise, sports and life with diabetes. After all, yoga practice can reduce stress, develop focus and discipline, and inspire a sense of well being. ⅔⅔

DANA HARITON

The Yin-Yang of Yoga and Good Sneakers

Dana Hariton is always on the move. She believes that having Type 1 diabetes correlates perfectly with having a Type A personality, which is evident when you see Dana pursue athletics with speed and focus.

Dana is a traveling runner and yogini, meaning that she has planted her sneakers and spirit down on terra firma in many lands. Besides running in her native New York City Marathon, she sped through one in New Zealand, and has also run in Kenya, India, Manila, Egypt, Peru and Panama. In fact, she has traveled to every continent except Antarctica. For Dana, a key factor about running is that all you need is a great pair of sneakers—and, naturally, an abundant supply of glucose gel and

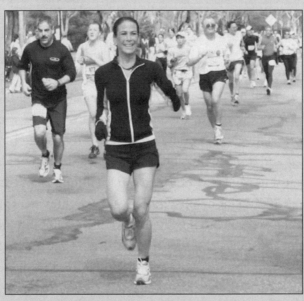

Dana Hariton

a CGM (Continuous Glucose Monitor)—and you are "good to go" for miles and marathons. In fact, Dana never leaves home without her sneakers. Working in the field of training and organizational development within corporations can be extremely stressful at times. When it gets too intense, Dana either sneaks off to the corner of her office and does a shoulder or head stand for ten minutes or goes out for run.

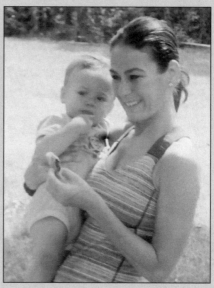

Mom Dana with precious Jack

Yoga has become an integral part of Dana's everyday life. It is something that helps calm down her Type-A energy and keeps her balanced and flexible physically, mentally and spiritually. Yoga is also the perfect "yin" accompaniment to her high "yang" activities of running and keeping blood sugars well managed.

In 2010, after painstakingly practicing tight control of her blood sugars, Dana gave birth to the apple of everyone's eye—healthy, young Jack Hariton McQuade, born August 21. Within a few months, Dana had Jack in his jogging stroller … and off they went to run in the park.

Dana volunteers her organizational skills to DESA and DIVABETICS whenever she has a spare minute from her busy days. As a certified diabetes coach (*www.balancelives.com*) she does her best to be a role model, educating and inspiring women. She particularly advises women to love and respect their bodies and the diabetes. Her view is that while diabetes certainly needs attention, you shouldn't judge yourself by the numbers you see on your glucose meter and A1C tests alone. Seek out help if you find yourself on the diabetes roller coaster, and never forget that you are in charge and can take control of your life and your diabetes. ✄

CHAPTER 9

Diabetes in the Wilderness
and the Water

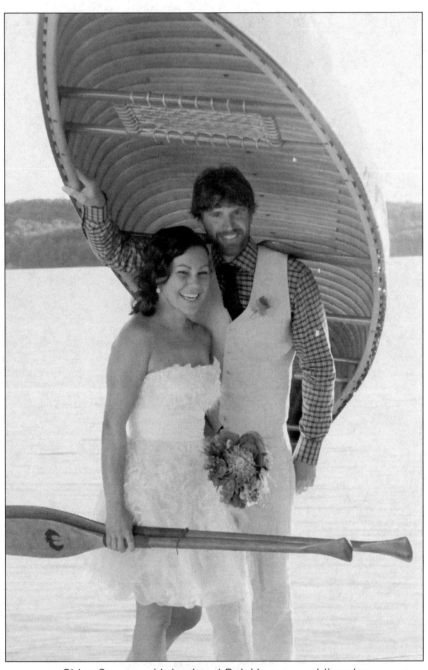

Chloe Steepe with husband Rob Vance, wedding day

CHLOE STEEPE

Connected In Motion

Chloe Steepe is "connected in motion" and flies on "slipstreams."
Connected In Motion (CIM) is a Canadian not-for-profit
diabetes organization that strives to connect, educate and inspire people
living with Type 1 by offering experiential diabetes education through
outdoor adventure and athletic pursuits.

And "slipstreams" (as defined by *Connected In Motion*) have several
applications: they can refer to the currents that produce reduced air
pressure and forward suction directly behind a rapidly moving person
with diabetes! Used as a verb, to "slipstream" can mean to ride this
current of a fast moving person with diabetes. Finally, it can simply
apply to the momentum that first created *Connected In Motion*.

Being "in the slipstream" happens for participants in the CIM events
when they gather together for weekends of athletics and good company.
As Chloe Steepe describes the experience:

*For one weekend we live in utter and complete diabetes bliss. We
live in a place where Dex4 glucose tabs flow freely from everyone's
pockets, where test strips on the floor can't be blamed on one person
alone, and where drinking juice in bed in the middle of the night
is normal, a place where others recognize the tunes of your pump
alarms, where you can lick blood off your finger without even a
sideways glance and where no one judges when you say you're "so*

high"! We draw up insulin at the dinner table, get excited over
straight lines on continuous glucose monitor graphs and for one
whole weekend we let our pump tubing hang loose.

That's what being in the *slipstream* is all about. Being a part of that
world for just a few short days is what keeps us cruising all year.

Steeped in Wanderlust

Chloe calls herself a "wander luster," and admits to an insatiable need to
keep her things in a backpack, pannier or barrel and hit the rivers, trails
and forests for as much of the year as physically possible.

I was curious when I heard this description. Wander luster? How
does a girl raised in downtown Toronto become an intrepid worldwide
wander luster? Chloe told me that she spent her childhood "pirouet-
ting" in ballet, "tumbling" in gymnastics and "spinning" in figure
skating. Circus school was also a major activity during elementary
school years, and she was quite the little twinkling star, breezing as light
as air on trapeze, walking the tightrope and tumbling. But all this fun
was secondary to horseback riding, which began when she was six years
old. Growing up as a "horsey kid," Chloe rode English and competed in
jumping and Eventing from grade school right through university.

Thinking back on her fifteen years of riding she remembers:

I think what I loved most about riding—aside from the horses and
friends—was getting out of the city. Growing up in downtown
urban Toronto, I looked forward to Friday nights when I could leave
school stresses behind and enter a whole other world—the barn.
At the barn, I had an entirely separate set of friends, routines and
priorities—much different from most other urban kids. Much to my
parents chagrin—after fifteen years, a couple of horses and countless
horseshow weekend—I think they wished I had chosen rec. soccer.
But I will always appreciate those years, the wonderful memories

and be thankful to them for providing such a privilege.

During high school, Chloe also played soccer, softball and ice hockey. Of course this little dynamo was a straight A student, too. As she puts it, "I loved school and always loved organizing, color coding and having everything in its place, which I think helps anyone to do well in school."

The Trip of a Lifetime

When Chloe was eighteen, during the summer before

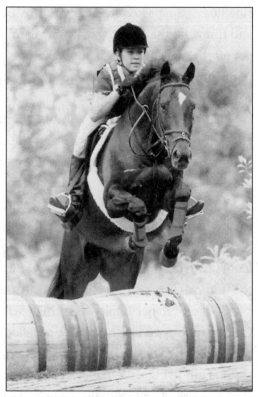

See Chloe jump

her senior year in high school, she spent an entire month in the Galapagos Islands in Ecuador completing biology credits.

During that month, however, she became really ill—lost thirty pounds in three weeks, had blurred vision, extreme thirst, infections and was peeing "all the time." Still, she was having the greatest time with twenty classmates; this was the trip of a lifetime! There was no way she was going home early. Instead, she completely convinced herself that she was having a reaction to malaria medications or that she had contracted a parasite or tropical disease of some sort. Since many of her classmates had experienced some form of illness too, she just figured she had it worse.

By the end of the month, Chloe was in rough shape—emaciated, dehydrated and constantly dizzy—but still having fun! On the plane ride home she passed in and out of consciousness a number of times and threw up the entire way from Miami to Toronto. When she finally got off the plane in Canada she was almost unrecognizable. Her mother burst into tears! But Chloe somehow managed to convince mom to take her home and not the hospital.

During the night Chloe awoke thinking she was having a heart attack. Pain shot down her arms and she could see her heart pounding in her skinny little chest. She was rushed to the emergency room where the doctors knew almost immediately that she had Type 1 diabetes.

"I will *always* remember that moment because I thought they were totally crazy," Chloe remarked. "Not *diabetes*?!!—that old fat person's disease? That was all I knew about diabetes at the time. I was sure they hadn't listened to a word I had said about my travels, the Amazon and the tropical diseases I was sure I had. Turns out, they were right!"

By the time her final year of high school started up in September, Chloe had learned much about the challenges, methods of treatment, as well as many of the nuances and subtleties that are part of the deal that comes with living with diabetes.

She learned that we diabetics hold the baton of conducting our lives in a healthy, fulfilling, hopefully uncomplicated way.

My Mom now jokes that diabetes was the best thing that could have happened to our family—in terms of awareness, knowledge and education in all things health and nutrition related. For me, my diagnosis changed my career path. Instead of going to veterinary college, I decided to pursue a degree in Physical and Health Education. I was inspired to learn more about my body and the way it works, as well as understand nutrition and physiology. I also wanted to pursue a career that would allow me to be active as part of my job. I quickly learned the importance of physical activity as a tool for good diabetes management. Diabetes is what gives me the incentive to get out and exercise even when I am feeling lazy.

It pushes me to prove to myself that I CAN *push my physical limits if I choose to.*

Through diabetes Chloe has met an incredible population of people who live with diabetes. They are strong, inspired, motivated, passionate, caring, generous and active. It has inspired her to reach out to others in the diabetes community and has sparked the creation of *Connected In Motion.*

> *Diabetes is not* WHO *I am, but it has helped to shape the person I have become.–* Chloe

On the Road

Chloe and Rob Vance, her "Type 3" partner, went on a two-month unsupported cycle tour of New Zealand's South Island as part of four months of travel through New Zealand and Australia. During this adventure of trying something she had never done before, cycling, Chloe chartered a course of "experiential diabetes education." Although she had learned the basic tools of diabetes management when she was in the hospital back home in Toronto, no one seemed to be able to answer questions about where to store an insulin pump in a wet suit while surfing, or how to keep insulin cold during two months on the road. But, that basic training encourage her to be confident in taking her diabetes into her own hands, at least for a while, and sharpened her skill to figure things out on the road, dealing with problems as they arose.

That bike trip taught her:

- How much basal rate reduction is needed for two hours of surfing
- That eating an entire kilo of irresistible strawberries as you pick them from the patch will have an impact on blood sugar

- The surge of adrenaline after being chased by an angry bull on a gravel road has a big impact on blood sugars
- In order to change a flat bicycle tire in a remote area, it is important to have stable blood sugars and a clear mind
- Climbing mountains, surfing, hiking, canoeing, camping, kayaking and cycling all have their own particular lesson to teach about the behavior of blood glucose levels.

Most of all, Chloe says,

Even more than spectacular sunrises and sunsets, breathtaking scenery around every bend in the road, shimmering blue lakes and lush rainforests, it was the realization that stemmed from my experiential diabetes education while traveling, that I think will have the greatest lasting impact. By respecting diabetes and its daily demands, it allows me to travel, get on a bike and cycle the South Island of New Zealand or head into the wilderness for weeks on end to canoe, hike and explore at will.

Connected in Motion to the World Around Her

Besides her buoyant energy and blithe spirit, I wondered what Chloe's credentials were that allowed her to embark on and claim responsibility for something as bold as CIM.

What I discovered was that Chloe holds a Bachelor's degree in education, along with another degree in outdoor experiential education; that she has completed an eighty-hour course which certified her as a Wilderness First Responder; she is a swift water rescue technician, a Nahanni River guide, and a flat water canoe instructor. Since 2004 she has guided extended canoe and raft trips in Ontario, Quebec, the Yukon and Northwest Territories. She has embarked on outdoor adventures throughout Europe, Central and South America, and, as we know, in Australia and New Zealand.

Whether the spark ignited on her first five-day canoe trip or her first mountain peak, she feels that being outdoors and self-propelled by her own energy and efforts and simplifying life to basic needs—food, water, shelter and warmth, slowing down and being observant—is what gives Chloe a refreshing, invigorating and fantastic feeling and the added bonus of improved blood sugars.

Being active outdoors gives us time to ponder and
appreciate what we have to be thankful for.– Chloe

Chloe reflects on how lucky she has been to have the unconditional support of her parents, especially at times when she has made unconventional decisions. Their encouragement and guidance have afforded her opportunities to travel, explore and discover her passions, as well as the freedom she needed to pursue them.

About her dreams for the next adventure, Chloe has her sights set on cycling South America as well as the entire West Coast of Canada, Inuvik to Vancouver. Aside from adventures on the road, she also hopes to paddle a canoe across Canada. No matter what she is doing, she hopes to be healthy, happy and active. "To love what I do and to do what I love. To continue building *Connected In Motion* into a strong organization helping thousands of people across Canada and around the world connect with one another to educate and inspire each other to take control of their diabetes."

Diabetes Exposed

One way Chloe likes to define herself is as a "multi-faceted dabbler in all things athletic and outdoorsy." Although this may sound idyllic for some, there have been and are occasional obstacles along her path— dehydration induced hyperglycemia on long hikes, spoiled insulin on glorious sunny hot canoe trips, frozen and shattered pump tubing while dog sledding at minus forty degrees, meters that are too hot or too cold to test bg's, or fingers that are too numb to bleed, to name a few.

Chloe offers "Strategies for Diabetes Exposure"—some solutions to life in nature with diabetes that she has learned through her experiential diabetes education:

- Become a master at packing. The better you are at cramming things into small spaces, the less likely you will have to choose between socks or infusion sets. Submit to the fact that your personal pack will look like a drug store.
- Start seeing double. Bring at least double the amount of supplies you need for the duration of the trip and bring a backup system or two. On any kind of wilderness adventure Chloe brings a backup pump, her old insulin pen as well as syringes. She has all her pump settings written out in case she has to change to a new pump. About meters—always bring two or three in addition to extra batteries and TONS of strips.
- Get proofed. Waterproof, sand proof and dirt proof your supplies. Keep things in small waterproof "sealine" bags (these can be purchased at most outdoor stores) even if you don't intend on getting wet.
- Sweet-talk your friends. Kindly ask fellow paddling, climbing, hiking partners to stash a (small, compressed, and well organized!) pack of back up supplies into the bottom of their pack for you, just in case. Batting eyelashes and/or offering to buy a pint after the trip often gets the job done. On remote northern expeditions where help is days away and the potential to be separated from out boats and gear is high, keep Dex4, bars, syringes, insulin, a meter and strips on your person in a PFD life jacket at all times. Never keep all your eggs in one basket.
- Embrace your inner squirrel. Squirrel away granola bars, fruit-to-go bars, Dex4, jelly beans and more in every pack, jacket

pocket, canoe and lifejacket, so carbs are always on board. Nothing is more annoying than having to ask the entire group to pull over while you fumble through eight packs trying to find a juice box. Remember to un-squirrel all of your goodies at the end of the day if you are camping in bear country.

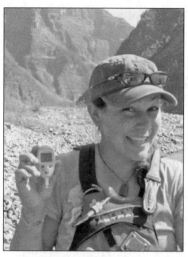

On kayak trip, with trusty glucose meter

- Be as meticulous about your insulin as Goldilocks was about her porridge. Keep it cozy warm but not too warm in the winter months. I like to keep my insulin and meter in two Spibelts under my parka while camping, snowshoeing, skiing, and dog sledding, or in a small insulated pack with a warm thermos on extended expeditions. Keep it cool but not too cool in the summer months. On a canoe trip, I keep some insulin buried deep within a canoe pack or barrel, and am conscious of keeping it out of direct sunlight and heat as best I can. I use a Frio for my insulin as well, dunking the sack in the lake or river to refresh it every once in awhile.

- Be prepared. Be confident. Be creative. Have a backup plan for your backup plan. Ensure you are well prepared with the material things before you set out. After that it's all about having the confidence to know that you can manage problems as they arise, troubleshoot and make good decisions.

- Get the inside scoop. Connect with people with diabetes who have been where you are going or have successfully done what you intend to do. Better yet, head out on a trip with them. There are a handful of organizations around the globe that provide these types of opportunities and experiences.

• Get outside!

⚜

Obviously, Chloe is a young woman who strives to face each challenge life throws. "Face it, challenge it back and overcome it," she proclaims. And this attitude marks her take on diabetes, too. She faces it head on, understanding that for now it is something she can't make go away but that it is manageable and many options, incredible technology and medical support are available.

Speaking with Chloe and having the pleasure of being in her company, I see how the little girl who rode horses and went to circus school has grown into a vivacious prime mover, one who sets high standards for all of us in the Sisterhood of Diabetes. ⚜

MONICA PRIORE

Swimming for the Children

In 2008 Paula Harper and I were invited to attend the First Italian Diabetes and Physical Activity Global Forum in Villasimius, Sardinia. There is no direct route to Sardinia from the east coast of the U.S. But once you set foot on this scenic and magical island you'll want to linger for a long visit.

The purpose of the forum, organized by a diabetologist from Naples, Dr. Gerardo Corrigliano, was a call to arms supported by the Italian Ministry for Health, to incorporate exercise as a therapeutic prescription for treatment of diabetes and for those at risk. One task of the meeting was to establish guidelines and initiatives to further promote this concept and create a consensus document to put into play on a national level in hospitals, diabetes clinics and diabetes organizations. In other words, for patients to be given prescriptions to show up at healthcare centers to learn and practice how to run, power walk, cycle, fence, and swim and play team sports. The emphasis of the prescriptions was to highlight to patients the importance of physical activity as an integrate part of excellent diabetes management.

The attendees at the forum were doctors, exercise physiologists, clinicians and patients. Sardinia was the perfect venue to explore sport and exercise opportunities. It is conducive to hiking, running in the hills, horseback riding, rowing, kayaking, swimming, sailing and naturally, playing soccer.

Monica's Presentation

One of the key speakers at the forum was Monica Priore, a patient. Monica was chosen because of the highly inspirational effect her life with diabetes has had on breaking down barriers and inspiring children with diabetes.

Monica was diagnosed with Type 1 diabetes in 1981 at age five at a clinic in Brindisi, Italy, not far from her home in nearby Mesagne. She has vague memories of being at the clinic and thinking it was a game with people dressed all in white, taking blood from her and giving her injections. She didn't understand that this "game" would be played for the rest of her life.

Monica was an active child, but in the 1980s in Italy exercise and sports was not looked upon favorably for people with diabetes, especially young children, because it would throw their blood sugars off kilter. But by the time Monica was eleven, she started playing volleyball and joined a team at school.

In Italy there are several levels of sports participation. One is general activity without competition, in other words "playing for fun." To join this level, one must present a doctor's note from a family physician. For competitive sports that engage in matches and races, it is required to go through several physical examinations and present written documentation from a sports physician. The certification granted is valid for one year.

In Monica's case, while the doctor did not certify her to play competitive volleyball because of diabetes, she continued to play with all her heart and soul at the recreational level until she was eighteen. Still, Monica harbored feelings of anger and disappointment that she did not qualify to play volleyball at the higher competitive level. And so what did she do? She jumped in the water and started to swim.

The Free Style of Swimming

A sport can groom passion, excitement, strength and a sense of freedom. Swimming accomplished all of these attributes for Monica. The more

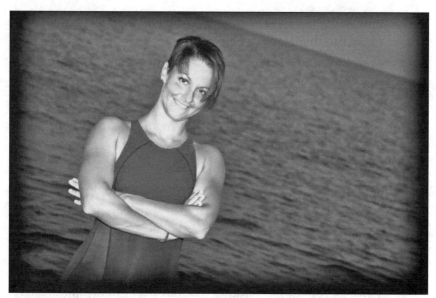

Monica Priore

she practiced and trained, her swimming skills grew. She also began to understand that she could excel at a sport even though she had diabetes—quite a revelation for this courageous young woman who, in the beginning, had no support for pursuing her belief.

As her confidence grew, so did her sense that people with diabetes are capable of achieving whatever goals they reach for. She knew that those in the clinical diabetes community in Italy at that time disagreed. They still believed that too much activity might be dangerous or make it difficult to manage diabetes. For her part, however, Monica determined to demonstrate that diabetes and exercise go hand in hand. It became clear to her that she must direct her diabetes and not let diabetes direct her.

Swimming became a major facilitator for this. She learned so much about how to regulate her blood sugars through documenting her activities, researching and studying, speaking with diabetologists and in essence using herself as a guinea pig. Controlling the excursions of low and high blood glucose levels that occurred as part of her experimental phase, Monica worked hard to close the gaps and balance blood sugars. She now refers to diabetes as a constant presence in her life. "If it were not this way, I would forget him and that means I would not be able to control him," she says.

Since taking up her mission, Monica has won over thirty-seven swimming medals: nine gold, eleven silver and sixteen bronze. The most prestigious among them are:

- An honorary medal received from the president of Italy, Giorgio Napolitano, to recognize Monica on her Capri-Sorrento crossing
- Freestyle 400 meter bronze in 2007
- Freestyle 200 meter silver in 2009
- Participation in the National Masters Championships 400, 800 and 1200 meter swims.
- In the Italian Masters Championships, Monica was honored to compete with former professional athletes.

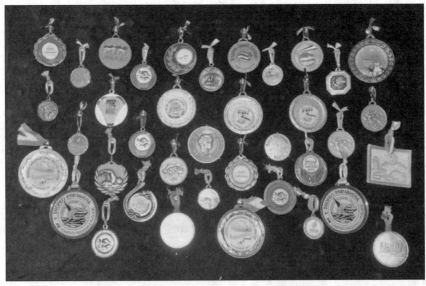

Some of Monica's awards

Although freestyle is her main swimming stroke, she also participates in high-level mixed styles in some competitions.

Aside from long hours of training for races and swimming events Monica works a full time job as a secretary, but hopes that one day soon she will work in the diabetes community with Type 1s as an advocate for physical activity.

The Presence of a Hero

When I met Monica in Sardinia at the diabetes forum I was captured by the way she carried herself—with dynamism, style and the sophistication that only a young Italian woman can capture. When called to the podium at the conference, there were cheers and applause from the medical professionals in the audience. *Brava! Monica!* they sang out. Monica had proven to these clinicians that yes, indeed, a person with diabetes has the ability to push the limits and grab the brass ring.

Monica was at the conference to talk about her recent success completing a swim in the rough and dangerous waters of the Straits of Messina. She took on this challenge to demonstrate the capabilities of a person with Type 1 diabetes. The swim itself was only 5K, which took about one hour and forty minutes, but the strong and sometimes dangerous currents in the Straits made this swim a huge victory, and one that had never been attempted by a person with Type 1 diabetes.

Medical doctors in Italy studied Monica's accomplishment as an example to encourage patients to become more physically active. It was after that successful swim, followed by the forum in Sardinia, that Monica realized that she had become a role model for others with diabetes, and especially for children. Her great desire was, and continues to be, to inspire children and their parents to believe and trust in themselves and know that if she accomplished her goals with swimming, they too can do whatever they choose in life.

Monica continues to work tirelessly to reach out to the diabetes community in Italy as someone who says, "*Lo facto Io, se poi fare anche tu!*" (I did it and so can you!) As part of her heartfelt devotion to this mission she challenged herself in 2010 to attempt an 18.5 km. open sea swim from Capri to Meta di Sorrento.

About Sardinia and Diabetes

Sardinia, the second largest island off Italy's coast is situated across from Corsica and north of Tunisia. It is a place that, after thousands of years of invasion and occupation, has remained fiercely independent and self sustaining. Its people say "*Sono Sardo, poi Italiano*" ("First I am Sardinian, then Italian"). The natural beauty of the island woos one to linger and explore the miles of crystalline coast, rugged caves and coves, ancient stone towers, the silken sand and blue-green waters of the Mediterranean Sea. The rough hewn mountainous center of the island shimmers with olive groves, grapes, herds of goats, small villages and countless sheep. The island is truly a paradise.

Besides being interesting and beautiful, there are a couple of medical mysteries about Sardinia that have scientists scratching their heads. Sardinia claims its place as one of the top "blue" spots for longevity, where people live to be well over 100, and next to Finland, it has the highest instances of Type 1 diabetes in the world. They seem so opposite, Sardinia and Finland. What is it that makes these geographically and culturally diverse places so susceptible to Type 1 diabetes? Theories, hunches and numerous studies abound, but facts remain rather inexplicable. One theory is that a common genetic root, the Y chromosome specifically, may have traveled from Northern Europe to Sardinia from as long ago as the Ice Age. Another theory is that unusual dietary patterns cause higher than normal prevalence of an inborn defect in metabolism of vitamin D that interferes with absorption.

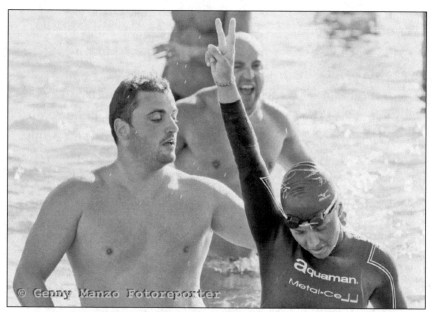

Monica's triumph after a perilous swim

Alessandro Capri, a fellow Type 1 athlete from Firenze (Florence, Italy), translated Monica's description of this swim:

The open waters of the Gulf of Naples had fierce weather conditions the morning of the swim. The winds were strong with 50-55 cm high waves. I'd have to postpone my task. I was told that it was highly dangerous to attempt the 18.5 km swim from Capri to Meta di Sorrento in such unfavourable conditions. But I had to do it. There was no turning back. I had no choice but to honour the commitment I had made. How could I even think of disappointing the many parents and especially the diabetic kids who came from all over Italy to support me in my task? They were on the beach waiting for me at Meta di Sorrento. I had trained rigorously during the four months leading up to this day. After my first success of crossing of the Straits of Messina, I wanted to do another bigger, more challenging swim to carry the message to all

Sardinia and Food

With diabetes we "are what we eat." Therefore, I must mention a word about food in Sardinia.

A meal is never rushed in Italy, especially in Sardinia where the attitude is for slow paced enjoyment. I consider the Sardinian diet to be the perfect balance of healthy nutrients, especially for people with diabetes, as it consists of fresh locally grown foods prepared in a simple style that incorporates olive oil, lemon, herbs and garlic to compliment dishes.

Meals are served in small courses usually with a pasta or soup first, then the main course of the day (fish served with local vegetables), followed by a simple refreshing salad to aid digestion at the end.

Desserts are primarily a delectable fresh sheep's milk cheese and fruit picked from nearby trees or berry patches. While it is impossible to duplicate the flavors and tastes, I brought back some simple and wonderful recipes from my time there. Here's one to enjoy.

Zucchini with Mint
Makes 6 servings

1 ½ Tbs. olive oil

3 scallions, thinly sliced

2 lbs. local dark-green zucchini, cubed into large bite-sized pieces

Pinch of salt

3 Tbs. each: flat leaf parsley and mint, shredded

½ cup crumbled Ricotta Salata cheese (Ricotta Salata is aged ricotta cheese with salt added. It is easily found in any specialty cheese store. Many supermarkets now carry it also.)

2 sheets *pane carasau* ("Sardinian music bread." *Pane carasau* is a traditional Sardinian paper-thin flat bread that is known as "music bread" because the pieces are so thin they resemble sheets of music. It can be found at *www.gournetsardinia.com.*

Its crispness and rich olive taste is truly unique and delicious. Worth ordering if you cannot find it at a local Italian specialty grocer. You can substitute very thin crisp bread. An expression in Sardinia goes—"Eat *pane da musica* (music bread) and live to be *cent' anni* (100 years)!"

Warm oil in skillet over medium high heat. Add scallions and sauté for 1 minute. Add zucchini, parsley and salt. Lower heat a little and cook, stirring occasionally, for about 5 minutes until zucchini is crisp tender.

Add mint and cheese. Toss. Cook for 1 minute. Serve over each piece of music bread.

APPROXIMATE NUTRITIONAL VALUE: ½ cup zucchini mixture with 1/3 piece of bread = 160 cal, 5 fat grams, 7 grams protein, 22 carb grams

people with diabetes that if you learn to manage your condition in the best way possible for you, nothing is precluded. Therefore I couldn't think about not attempting this swim. I was committed and passionate about it. It was too important for me.

I dropped myself into the water at ten o'clock in the morning and started to face the high waves and sea streams as onlookers watched incredulously. I swam in the open waters for six and a half hours. During this time I had several problems but I never thought to interrupt my task. I approached the support boat every forty minutes to check blood glucose to decide if I needed sugar or nutrition. The extreme wave conditions obliged me to stop swimming occasionally because of seasickness but a voice inside me kept saying: "Don't give up." I had to take a pill for nausea and then I went on swimming. In the blurry distance, I spotted crowds of people on the beach at Meta di Sorrento. Despite my discomfort and agony I couldn't help but smile. By the end of the swim I had swam for 21 km instead of the original 18.5 ones because of the powerful tidal stream.

When I emerged from the water the emotions of the crowd were so powerful that many people, including myself, cried. I understood that my goal was the same as everyone who had come to support this effort. There were so many people and reporters present. I felt exhausted but so very joyful. Somehow a bright smile came over me. People asked me where I was finding the force to smile. Even if I was very tired, I was smiling to all. My goal had been achieved! Not only the accomplishment of succeeding at a sport but also the human goal. I know this because after that memorable day, many diabetic children and parents sent me so much mail thanking me for what I did for them. They understood that you don't have to stop yourself in front of adversity. They consider me an example to follow. This is a great responsibility for me, so I hope and pray to never disappoint them.

Brava! Monica! Congratulations on your strong and unselfish work. We are so proud of you. You truly are an inspiration in the Sisterhood of Diabetes. ༀ

CHAPTER 10
Academics and Advocates

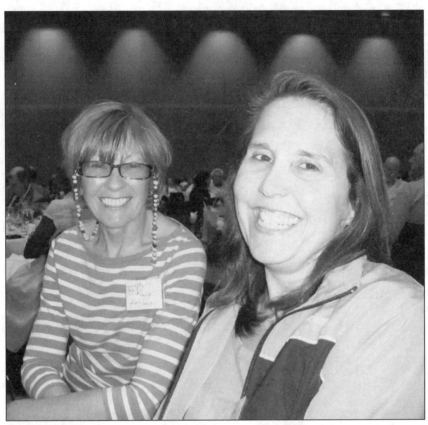
Sheri Colberg-Ochs (right) and author at conference, Raleigh, N.C.

DR. SHERI COLBERG-OCHS

She Does It All!

The Sheri Colberg-Ochs you may know about is a scholar and prolific writer in the field of diabetes, and particularly diabetes and exercise. She is the diabetic athlete with a PhD in exercise physiology, the one we in the "business" go to when we can't figure out answers to complicated questions about blood sugars and sports. Sheri has hiked to the top of the mountain in her area of expertise. To give you an overview of some of her many accomplishments:

- She has written and published eight books since 2001(some have been translated into multiple languages)
- Has authored seven book chapters
- Has written over two hundred articles
- Produces a blog and two websites
- She is the American Diabetes Association representative for the National Physical Activity Plan launched in May 2010.
- Serves as a member of the newly formed ADA Prevention Committee
- Serves as a member of the American College of Sports Medicine's Pronouncements Committee
- First author of the joint American College of Sports Medicine/ADA position stand on Type 2 diabetes and exercise

- She has authored two chapters on exercise/physical activity for the American Association of Diabetes Educators guidelines book
- A BOD member and regular contributor to the *DESA Challenge* magazine

These luminous pearls comprise the necklace that Sheri has strung for herself over the forty-plus years she has lived with Type 1 diabetes.

Embracing the Power of Knowledge and Movement

Sheri spent most of her childhood years traveling around the country, as her family moved from Missouri to Oregon to Kansas to Oklahoma to Colorado to Minnesota before finally settling down in Atlanta for seven years. As a smart, tough kid, Sheri learned to cope with the impermanence of constant moving and starting over by turning to books, and by becoming a strong athlete.

A formidable student, achieving a 4.0 average throughout school, Sheri was named valedictorian in high school. Her success in school encouraged her to continue to high levels of academic achievement. She also became an athlete.

As a child, Sheri always felt good when she was active, and this appreciation of energy and healthiness led her in her adult life to become an exercise physiologist and researcher in diabetes and exercise, and in the prevention of diabetes complications through physical activity.

Her first love in sports was swimming, and that remains right up to the present. Swimming came naturally to Sheri, who thinks back to when she was a kid and spent every spare minute in the pool. (One of her three sons is like that too, she notes. "It must be in the genes.")

Without the support of more recently developed tools such as a bg meter or CGM or pump—which probably kept her from being as competitive as she would have like to be—Sheri still knew for sure was that when she exercised or played sports she felt much better and more in control of her diabetes. Her mother was not so keen on her tomboy ways, however, but despite her mother's hesitancy, Sheri, with her dogged determination, played on soccer teams throughout high school, in addition to swimming, tennis, gymnastics and volleyball. In her "spare" time, she played racquetball. And if that wasn't enough for this "jack of all sports," in senior year of high school she started lifting weights.

Remarkably, even without a bg meter, she made it through her younger years without a single low blood sugar reaction or hypoglycemia, and was never hospitalized for anything related to diabetes, not even DKA. But, as she says, she always took her insulin, even though it was not possible to adjust doses to match blood glucose levels back then.

Once Sheri arrived at college in California, a new sport impassioned her—football. It became *her* sport, as well as her job to help pay for school.

I worked for four years as student equipment manager for the Stanford University football team, a Pac 10 Division 1 school. This meant I had to go to all of the practices, set up the fields for the coaches, help with drills and put everything away afterwards. I went to almost all of the games with the exception of some of the away games for the first three years. I loaded and unloaded gear and helped during the games. It was a very physically active job and I loved every minute of it. I remember a coach telling me the first year that I threw like a girl and he taught me how to spiral a football just the right way. I can still do it! I was the first and only woman equipment manager for the Stanford team from 1981-85. But, my real claim to fame was being the first woman head student equipment manager of a Division 1 team. Yes, I was a jock.

Sheri will always be a jock … as I see it. These days it's swimming (of course), conditioning machines, weight training, walking, hiking and biking.

Family, Home and Work Life

Sheri and her husband and best friend, Ray Ochs, have a busy family life raising three boys, Alex, 16, Anton, 14 and Ray J, 11. Spending time with them is one of the greatest and most profound joys of her life.

Before her first pregnancy, Sheri took part in a study looking at the effects of counseling on prevention of birth defects in infants of Type 1 mothers. (She admits doing this mainly for the free bg monitoring strips.) With this, she also learned the valuable lesson of how to control bg's with great precision before becoming pregnant. The end result was three completely uncomplicated pregnancies, and three healthy children.

During pregnancy Sheri found it easier to control her blood sugars since there was no dealing with those monthly hormonal "meltdowns" that profoundly affect insulin action; the increase in insulin resistance was consistent and thus easier to manage. In 1993, before her first pregnancy, she also stopped all caffeine intake so that there would not be any caffeine present in utero. She never went back to caffeine, except for what is present in the chocolate she eats—which is usually a handful of dark chocolate almonds—most days.

Sheri's life is rich with family, teaching, research, writing, lecturing, exercise and sports. Today she works in the academic environment as a professor at Old Dominion University in Virginia, teaching graduate and undergraduate level sports nutrition and exercise physiology. She is an adjunct professor of internal medicine at Eastern Virginia Medical School, director of exercise physiology for Insulite Laboratories, and executive director of the Lifelong Exercise Institute, which she founded.

Sheri still manages to find time to give back to the diabetes community with copious amounts of volunteer work. She lectures about healthy lifestyle, answers peoples' online questions about diabetes on her websites: *www.shericolberg.com*, *www.lifelongexercise.com* and on *www.AllExperts. com*. For the American Diabetes Association and the American College of Sports Medicine, she serves on a number of committees on diabetes and exercise. Decidedly, it is important to Sheri to use her knowledge and expertise to help people live long and healthy lives, and to exercise safely and effectively.

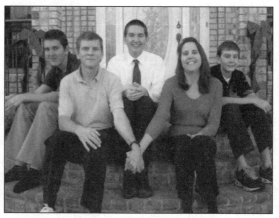

Sheri Colberg-Ochs and family

The Light in the Tunnel Gets Brighter

Sheri was diagnosed in 1968 during what she and others have called the "dark ages" of diabetes care, Imagine a feisty, teary-eyed little four year old telling her mommy to "practice more" in giving shots to an orange until she learned how to "do it better." Seems her mom had been following hospital instructions of injecting an orange as a teaching tool so she would be able to inject little Sheri's arm with insulin. As it happened, when the time came to switch from the orange to the delicate skin of a four year old, the shot ricocheted back since the child's arm was much easier to inject that the tough skin of an orange.

The face of diabetes has changed greatly in the more than forty years since then. The diabetes population has grown too large and too fast, unnecessarily in some cases, and Sheri sadly witnesses this unfortunate turn of events.

Too many people are overweight. Too many children are being diagnosed with Type 2 diabetes. Too many children are being diagnosed with Type 1 diabetes. But, as a powerful and highly respected force in the world of diabetes, Sheri speaks out to advocate the importance of a healthy lifestyle. With her credentials, experience, passion and drive, people listen.

Sheri holds great hope about finding a cure:

I am in the diabetes research world and privy to a lot of what is being investigated. One of my colleagues at Eastern Virginia Medical School has been researching, for years, ways to make the pancreas regenerate. His techniques, combined with some immune system modulation, will likely cure Type 1 diabetes. Type 2 will be harder, but I'm working on solving that problem through lifestyle change messages.

At Children With Diabetes conferences today, one can see different age groups from toddlers to teens wearing their insulin pumps without fear or embarrassment. These kids know the feeling of a "low," and they have been educated in how many carb grams they need to stop downward excursions.

In 2011, when I was speaking with a group of the ten- and twelve-year-old "tweeners," we were comparing pump colors and brands. It all seemed so normal and natural. But there was a level of bitter sweetness. On the one hand, the kids are so smart about their diabetes—fortunately insulin infusion pumps have always been here for them—and on the other hand, it is harsh and regrettable that they have diabetes at all.

Thanks, Superwoman!

Science, technology, research and education are all vital components in the mix of making diabetes management safe and inspired. But it's people like Sheri Colberg-Ochs who nudge the process along, keeping it in our faces. Without her insight, brilliance and drive there surely would be more obstacles in the way of the wheels of progress. She feels that anything in life is possible to achieve if you set your mind to it and …

Diabetes should never be your excuse for not reaching for the stars. Always live your life to the fullest, being mindful of diabetes, of course, and keep diabetes in the proper perspective. Having diabetes has been a great incentive to have direction and determination in all areas of my life. I am definitely an overachiever and have been my entire life. I often act like Superwoman and see how many things I can handle at once (I wrote two books simultaneously two years running, and five books total in two and a half years.) Most of the time I don't have any trouble handling it as long as I can get enough sleep and continue to work out consistently. If I didn't exercise and stay in shape, I probably wouldn't have the energy to get anything done. I set my own workout schedules and allow myself to do easier workouts on "tired" days and look at it as a lifelong commitment, so I can be healthy for myself and my family and avoid diabetic complications. I feel privileged to make my health a priority.

And we in the Sisterhood of Diabetes feel privileged to have Superwoman Sheri as one of our muses.   ⅋

Her Books

Exercise and Diabetes: A Clinicians Guide, ADA Books, 2013.
Diabetes-Free Kids, Muddy Paws Press, 2012.
The Diabetic Athlete's Handbook, Human Kinetics, 2009.
Diabetes? No Problema! Da Capo Press Life Long Books, 2009.
Matt Hoover's Guide to Life, Love and Losing Weight, Skyhorse Publishing, 2008.
50 Secrets of the Longest Living People with Diabetes, Marlowe & Company/Da Capo Books, 2007.
The Science of Staying Young, McGraw-Hill, 2007.
The 7-Step Diabetes Fitness Plan, Marlowe & Company, 2006.
The Diabetic Athlete, Human Kinetics, 2001.

Websites

Sheri Colberg: *www.shericolberg.com*
Lifelong Exercise Institute: *www.lifelongexercise.com*

BRANDY BARNES

She Turned Diabetes into a Gift

When I met Brandy at the first "Weekend for Women" conference she organized in Raleigh, North Carolina, in 2010, where I had the privilege to teach tai chi sessions, I thought she was very cool. Her keen awareness of the value of physical activity for women with diabetes was demonstrated with a variety of fun and interesting exercise protocols such as yoga, Zumba, belly dancing and tai chi. Since that first conference, even more activities have been added to programs. Health walks are now part of her *DiabetesSisters* conferences. They are another way to encourage women to participate in regular physical activity. The walks are also meant to increase awareness of the unique challenges faced by women with diabetes.

Brandy Barnes told me something that really struck a chord in my Type 1 psyche. She said "Do you view your diabetes as a burden or a gift? Life is ten percent what happens and ninety percent how you react to what happens. So, in fact, you do have a lot of control over your life." Brandy made the conscious decision to make her diabetes a gift and since her diagnosis in 1990, at age fifteen, she has taken her gift and opened a "gift shop" with it.

In 2007, after living with diabetes for over seventeen years, Brandy discovered its purpose in her life. She set out with great enthusiasm to create an organization whose purpose is to serve women with diabetes around the world. Armed with a B.A. in psychology and a Master's in social work from the University of North Carolina at Chapel Hill, she got to work. For three years Brandy served as the tireless volunteer founder and CEO responsible for marketing, fund raising, bookkeeping, program development and management, website management and a long list of other administrative and day-to-day tasks. The mission of the organization has remained the same since the day it was launched: to provide a support system of useful and meaningful programs, encouragement, empowerment, education and services for all women with diabetes. In other words, to help women reach their full potential. As Brandy says, "An empowered and informed woman with diabetes is a healthy woman with diabetes."

The name of Brandy's creation is closely related to the subject of this book. Brandy's life work is a 501c3 international non-profit organization called *DiabetesSisters*. Please take a look at the website *www. diabetessisters.org* to be inspired by all the wonderful outreach projects Brandy and her ever-expanding team of volunteers have developed since starting out with just a dream, a concept and one volunteer in 2007.

Today *DiabetesSisters* offers annual conferences on both coasts of the U.S. It attracts support from major diabetes associated corporations such as Roche and Sanofi. Through these sponsorships, *DiabetesSisters* communicates national support groups, weekly blogs from women living with diabetes, "From the Experts" columns from dedicated health professionals who live with diabetes, and a Sister Match Program. These offerings and many others present opportunities for women with diabetes to connect.

Her Personal Hero
The little person who scurries about helping with many *DiabetesSisters* tasks and loves to tell everyone she meets that, "My mom has diabetes and she started *DiabetesSisters*," is none other than Summer Barnes, her six-year-old daughter. As Brandy says about Summer, "She is my hero!"

Summer is mature beyond her years and is very protective of her mother. When they walk or do Zumba or Wii Dance together, Summer always makes it her mission to be sure Brandy has her meter and snacks before they leave the house. Because she has been so involved with *DiabetesSisters*, Summer has learned more about diabetes than most adults. She understands how to identify symptoms of hypoglycemia and has rehearsed calling 9-1-1 in case of an emergency situation.

At a Step-Out Walk with the American Diabetes Association, Summer was upset to see team T-shirts that read STOP DIABETES. Because she is so immersed in the world of *empowering* women with diabetes, she thought "ridding the world of diabetes" was something offensive. She looked at her mom and said, "Mommy, do we have to walk with those people with the

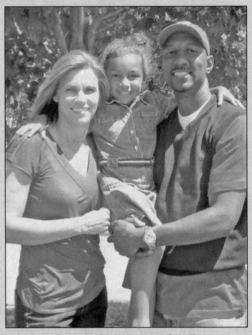

Brandy Barnes and family

shirts that say STOP DIABETES? That is mean. There's nothing wrong with having diabetes."

Life is quite busy these days as Brandy grows *DiabetesSisters*, serves on the North Carolina Diabetes Advisory Council and the American Diabetes Association Women's Work Group and raises her family. It wasn't all that long ago when Brandy was in grad school working on Type 1 and Type 2 research projects at the UNC Diabetes Care Center, then working as an Executive Sales Professional for Sanofi Corporation selling diabetes medications for six years. But her commitment to make the lives of women with diabetes better emerged as her clear mission and true calling. All of us, as women with diabetes, in the Sisterhood of Diabetes shout out a big THANKS to Brandy Barnes for her strength and dedication to improve the lives of women with diabetes. As Brandy says, "Everyone needs help at some time in their diabetes journey. No one, no matter how strong or fierce, can do diabetes alone!" 🦋

CHAPTER 11

The Upcoming Inspiration Generation

What happens when you are diagnosed with Type 1 diabetes? First of all, you are surprised if not shocked by this newcomer who has barged into your life. The initial days are spent learning what diabetes is, how to manage it and the many ways it can affect your body. It takes time, thought, patience and understanding to digest the fact that every morning you will wake up and you will have diabetes. Every night when you go to bed you will have diabetes. You eventually figure out how to negotiate with this "diabetes thing." You learn there are choices regarding how to steer this bold entity that has parked itself into your life's backyard without any intention of moving out.

Enter attitude and friendship. You can adopt a positive approach and understand that, if you make friends with diabetes, then "Life is just a bowl of cherries ...," as an old song first sung by Ethel Merman says. However, as you soon learn, it is also important to be aware that ten cherries contain fifteen grams of carbohydrate, which means that you need to count them into your daily food/insulin/exercise calculations in order to maintain good blood sugar numbers. At the same time, you learn that you can be the boss of your diabetes. The quicker you learn this, the easier it becomes to set an optimistic tone that will resound in many aspects of your life.

As a child or teenager, it is sometimes difficult to grasp the complexities of living with a chronic condition. Changing the way you eat, being aware of where your blood sugar numbers are going, especially during sports and exercise, juggling aspects of your social life and being strong and responsible enough to make decisions about your diabetes management are all part of growing up with diabetes.

The young women you will meet in this chapter were all diagnosed early in life and have learned to make diabetes their friend ... well ... most days ... to have that positive attitude about life which encourages one to dream and set high goals.

As a result of this commitment, they motivate, excel, even "sparkle," as they do their best to keep diabetes by their side as they snowboard, play basketball and soccer, sail, dance, row, run, mountain climb and speed skate.

For as long as diabetes is with us, there will be generations of inspiration and role models who inspire. The young women in this chapter will surprise and shine a light of promise. They take it upon themselves to accept the responsibilities of diabetes. As Elise Zevitz, one of the young athletes you'll read about in this chapter, says:

> *Diabetes is a lot like driving a car with a manual transmission. You have more control, more involvement and more responsibility, just like all the best sports cars!* ❧❧

Feet on the Floor ...
Wind in Her Sails

According to Chelsea Brown, she is currently "on the cusp of honeymoon." You might ask "Where did she go? Hawaii? The Caribbean? Paris? No, No and No. You see it is not that kind of honeymoon. It's the honeymoon phase of diabetes. According to the Juvenile Diabetes Research Foundation (JDRF), the term *honeymoon* or *remission phase* is a time period of weeks, months or sometimes years when, after diagnosis of Type 1 diabetes, blood glucose levels are brought under control and any existing beta cells recover temporarily and produce some insulin, thus keeping the need for injected insulin at a relatively low level.

Chelsea was sixteen at the time of her diagnosis of diabetes. Our interview took place in 2010 when she was eighteen and a senior in high school. At the time, she carried on with her busy life managing her diabetes attentively, studying for school, enjoying family and friends and sailing during the summers. She still does. She still moves through all activities of her life with the smooth and graceful rhythm of a dancer.

On Her Toes

Chelsea took her first dance class at age three and has never stopped moving to the beat. Hip-hop, ballet, jazz, contemporary, modern and pointe are the types of dance Chelsea studies, practices, performs and is passionate about.

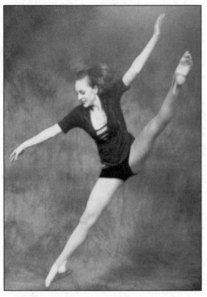

Chelsea Brown

She has been awarded the Maryland All-State dance title and the Emerging Artist Award. She dances with the Anne Arundel County Dance Ensemble and at her dance studio.

Dance can be rigorous. Some classes are half-hour blasts of non-stop energy, while others are long, stretchy two-and-a-half-hour sessions, but she keeps a close check on blood sugars, insulin dosage and snacks whenever appropriate, and drinks plenty of water.

During winter dance season, when rehearsals and performances occur almost every weekend, the excitement and nervousness before a performance can challenge her diabetes management. An adrenaline kick can elevate her blood glucose level. For Chelsea, the rule of thumb is not to exercise strenuously when blood glucose levels are over 250. That is also time to check for ketones in urine. But as Chelsea says, "The show must go on." By the end of a performance, blood sugar is usually back within normal range due to her careful insulin dosing and exercise combination.

Chelsea has made it a habit to alert teachers, friends and fellow dancers about her diabetes. She lets them know that sometimes it is necessary for her to stop to check her blood glucose or have a snack. Chelsea's go-to quick carbohydrate is cake gel. She shows her support "team" where she keeps it in case of emergency. This is a smart move on Chelsea's part. In fact, one of her friends, Matthew Stephens, carries a cake gel on his keychain. Another good friend, Daniel Fitzgerald, keeps a cake gel in his car, and both friends ask about her blood sugars if they haven't seen her check in a while.

Having friends and family who genuinely care for someone who has diabetes is a huge vote of love and support. They are affectionately known as our "Type 3s."

Sailing Away

When summer arrives, it is time for this dancer to relax her toes and head for the open waters of the Chesapeake Bay and the Magothy River in Maryland. After five years of studying and sailing at camp, she has worked her way up from the lowest level of Seaman III to Skipper (which means she is qualified to sail alone in windy conditions and to teach novice sailors). She has achieved recognition with both Future Instructor and Head Instructor awards for her skills, and is trained in CPR and First Aid. Although Chelsea is a qualified skipper, she usually has a fellow sailor on board, or her dad follows her in his motorboat for safety's sake.

After Chelsea's diagnosis, she and her mother reached out to local diabetes support groups and sailing programs for information. There was nothing available, so they launched their own research project to figure out the best methods to manage her diabetes and ensure her safety while sailing. They bought three waterproof bags to hold her juice, glucose meters and snacks. Two bags board the instructors' boats and one stays on Chelsea's boat. She also keeps a waterproof walkie-talkie on board in case of distress. She has not needed to test these measures yet, and hopefully never will, but at least she is prepared if a situation ever emerges.

As an advanced sailor and co-captain of the dance company, it is Chelsea's role and responsibility to portray a strong leadership position. Although diabetes can be a nuisance, Chelsea does not allow it to get in the way of carrying out her duties. She knows exactly how to maintain with the grace and lilt of a professional young woman who understands how to turn the beat around to accentuate the positive. Thanks, Chelsea Brown, for being part of the inspiration generation in the Sisterhood of Diabetes.   ✸

ASHLEY NAPEAR

Camper, Counselor, Coach

If it weren't for my diabetes, I never would have had the opportunity to go to CBC (Clara Barton Diabetes Camp for Girls with Diabetes) where I made so many friendships that I will keep for the rest of my life.

Camp had such a profound meaning for Ashley that she currently holds the position at The Barton Center as Clara Barton Camp Assistant Director. Ashley graduated from State University of New York (SUNY) Plattsburgh with a Bachelor of Arts degree in Criminal Justice,

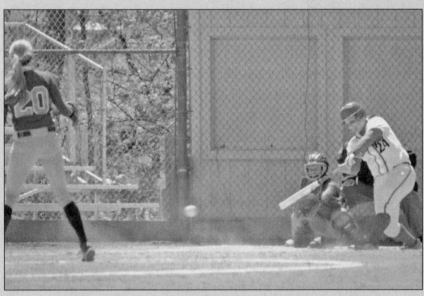

Ashley Napear batting against SUNY New Paltz in 2010

but her special dream is to find a career path in the field she loves most, diabetes camps. She has also earned an AS degree in Recreation, Parks and Leisure Studies from Northern Virginia Community College to help facilitate her dream of working in diabetes camps.

Being diagnosed with Type 1 diabetes as a young child turns life topsy-turvy. Fortunately several positive forces work to balance the burdens. One of these is summer camp, the place where children with diabetes not only have a ball, but learn about their diabetes and how to be responsible for it, meet and inevitably make "best friends" with other kids in the same situation. Camp is a new beginning every summer for a child or young person who lives with diabetes. It is important and potentially monumental. For Ashley Napear, camp has become her second home.

Playing on the Field of Life

Ashley worked as JV head coach for a local high school, and as assistant coach for the traveling softball team she played with back in middle school. These jobs kept her where she loves to be—on the field. But now she works at the place she had set her goals on many years ago, CBC, as assistant director.

Ashley advises everyone she meets is that "if they think they can't do sports because of diabetes, they should think again. Even though it can sometimes be difficult to control diabetes and play sports, regardless of the struggles, it is worth it one hundred percent!"

Thank you, Ashley Napear—camper, counselor and softball coach—for sharing your story and encouragement with all the sisters in our special "Camp" Sisterhood of Diabetes.   ᙠᙢ

Rebel with a Cause

A smile can be exceptionally revealing. A smile can say, "Welcome, here I am." It can also say, "I'm smart, gorgeous, strong, adventurous, funny and determined to make the world a better place for every person with diabetes." That's what Svati Narula's smile reveals.

Until she was nine years old, Svati did everything all the other kids did, which was, basically, have fun. But around the time of her ninth birthday, her mother—a nurse and diabetes educator—noticed that Svati was displaying some of the classic signs of Type 1 diabetes. Her instincts told her to use a glucometer testing meter and do a finger-stick blood test on her daughter. Then she stepped out of the room for a brief second. Svati saw the reading on the monitor and shouted to her mother "It says 464. That's normal right?"

Off they rushed to Children's Hospital where Svati was officially diagnosed with Type 1 diabetes.

The Fun of Running

At Svati's middle school there was something called the "fun run" test in gym class. This was a timed one-mile cross country run. Most of the kids dreaded it, but Svati took it seriously. Running made her feel good and she thrived on tracking her times. Her first one-mile run came in at 9:32. Soon it was 9:17. By the end of sixth grade 8:54 was a breeze for her. Each year her times improved and by eighth grade Svati was one of the best runners in school running a 7:14 mile.

Svati's insightful PE teacher was aware of her combination of discipline and talent, coupled with her joy in running. He encouraged her to join cross-country track in high school. She followed his advice, tried out and made the varsity squad as a freshman. It was the best decision she could have made in high school. Running gave her confidence and became a major learning experience in how to balance sports with diabetes.

Running into Politics

Every spring from 2002-2009, Svati led a team for the Juvenile Diabetes Research Foundation "Walk to Cure Diabetes" in Washington, DC, raising over $25,000 for the JDRF in those years. In high school she was recruited to write for the Health Central Network's Diabeteens website, where she kept a regular blog about issues that teenagers with diabetes face. Svati has participated in numerous research studies related to diabetes and has been a strong advocate for federal funding for more diabetes research. To this end, she has spoken at press conferences on Capitol Hill, given interviews on TV and met with senators and representatives about diabetes. She was a delegate at the JDRF Children's Congress in 2003 and in the summer of 2010 she worked as an intern

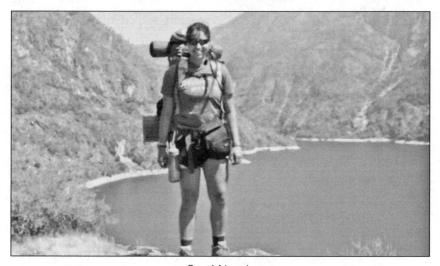

Svati Narula

Stress Release

Stress can have a disastrous effect on diabetes. It is not something that is emphasized much and maybe should be. What happened to Svati during the relay is not uncommon amongst diabetic athletes. Besides being physically prepared for an event by training and setting one's mind in racing gear, a certain background worry nags away about fluctuations in blood sugars, possible pump glitches and adequate fuel snacks. A few simple measures can help in reducing stress before an event: Close your eyes and take ten long slow and deep breaths, in through the nose and out through the mouth. Be sure your shoulders are loose and relaxed.

Hang like a rag doll. With feet wide apart, knees bent and body limp slowly hang the upper body to the left and drape over the thigh. Then come to center. Hang and relax. Don't forget to breathe slowly throughout. Repeat on right side. Do slowly and repeat several times until completely relaxed.

in the JDRF Government Relations office in DC. Through all this experience, Svati has gleaned an interest in public policy, especially health policy.

Student Athlete

During her freshman year at Dartmouth College, Svati joined crew, but decided to pull in the oars after a semester in the water, not because of the difficulty of the sport or of managing her diabetes but rather because the long hours required for training interfered with her studies. But she didn't leave sports completely. Far from it!

In 2009 she joined the Dartmouth Endurance Racing Team, which required running about twenty miles a week. She and six teammates ran the Race Across the State, a relay across the entire state of New Hampshire to raise money for a local Children's Hospital. This race proved particularly difficult for her because due to the difficulties of blood sugar management, she was stressed and feeling fatigued before running a step in this relay. Although she finished the race, incidents like this are what frustrate Svati the most about having diabetes.

Enter Insulindependence and Testing Limits

At about the same time she was trying her skills at other outdoor adventures—hiking, camping and skiing—Svati decided to step things up and train for a triathlon. That summer of 2009, while volunteering at the CWD (Children With Diabetes) conference in Orlando, she met an Ironman diabetic who told her about Insulindependence's (*www. insulindependence.org*) Triabetes club. Triabetes and the wider Insulindependence network led her to a community of Type 1s who test their athletic limits beyond what she thought possible. The mission of IN is to enable successful diabetes management through peer-supported fitness and adventure programs. This results in pinpointing the nuances and understanding more about being an athlete with diabetes.

Svati soon signed up to be a captain for IN's Testing Limits and has undergone leadership training hosted by IN to mentor children with diabetes, take them on wilderness expeditions and lead local fitness events. Read more about Testing Limits in Svati's September 17, 2010 article, "Testing Independency" in *Diabetes Health* magazine. (*www. diabeteshealth.com*)

Svati Narula is a leader and inspiration as she goes forth in life with that beautiful smile on her face, not accepting the status quo, but challenging it as a rebel with a cause for … the Sisterhood of Diabetes. ✣

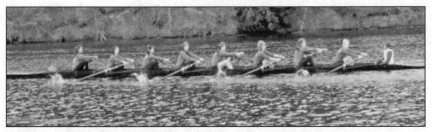

Svati "Strokewoman" at the stern

MAKYLA SEVER

Diabetes Ambassador

In 2008 at a Children With Diabetes conference at Disney Orlando, an athletic panel discussion for teens was hosted by Sports Central. One of the questions fielded to the panel of diabetic athletes was, "Do you remember the moment of your diabetes diagnosis?"

Will Cross (the first Type 1 to summit Mt. Everest), Doug Burns (Mr. Universe), Chris Dudley (long time professional basketball player) and Jay Leeuwenburg (pro-football player with the Indiana Colts), each described his clear recollections. When it came to Phil Southerland (founder and CEO of the Team Type 1 cycling team), he hesitated and thought hard for a moment, then said, "Well, my mom told me I cried, but it was probably because I needed my diaper changed. I was only seven months old at the time."

I was reminded of this story when I interviewed Makyla Sever who told me she didn't remember anything before taking shots. Makyla was diagnosed at seventeen months old. Today, this little dynamo from Winnipeg, Canada, is an athlete, singer and diabetes ambassador.

Makyla is an extremely ambitious girl who has not let diabetes infringe on her active lifestyle. She was selected as a youth ambassador for the JDRF (Juvenile Diabetes Research Foundation) in 2010. This meant volunteering at the Ride for Diabetes Research and participating in the JDRF Walk. Her assignment for the walk was to answer questions about diabetes, a job she took seriously and performed flawlessly. Makyla talked about the importance of funding for research, a subject close to her heart, as she and her family have raised thousands of dollars every year for this purpose.

Makyla volunteers at her school helping out kids who have disabilities. She aids a handicapped boy who is confined to a wheelchair and during recess she pushes a blind girl on the swings in the schoolyard.

Makyla's life is a busy one. She loves school and is an exceptional student. But after school, it's all about sports! She started playing ringette (girls ice hockey) at four years old, soon after she learned how to skate. Her older sister Lexi also plays ringette and following in her sister's footsteps Makyla has become a highly competi-

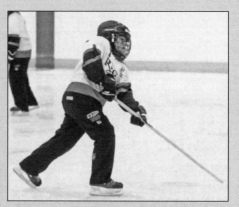

Makyla Sever controls the puck

tive player. She is also on a soccer team where she plays right down to the buzzer, giving it her *all* every minute of the game.

Makyla's parents have always emphasized that playing sports is an integral part of living a healthy life. Even though she is among the youngest athletes highlighted in this book, Makyla already understands the importance of taking good care of her diabetes. She stays away from eating too much candy, but admits that her favorite meal is mac and cheese … with tons of cauliflower and broccoli … and of course a little ice cream for dessert.

Having diabetes is not one of her favorite things in life, but as she says, "There is nothing I can do about it. Some kids have worse things and I am learning how to manage my diabetes better and better."

When I asked Makyla about her dreams for the future, she skipped a beat or two, then confidently came back with, "I want to be a famous singer. I love to sing and I'm not afraid to speak or sing in front of crowds of people. I also want to be a fashion model and design clothes. I also want to tell everybody about what it's like to have diabetes so they will do more to help. Maybe I'll write a book and be a teacher. I love to write new poems and songs." When we talked about a cure for diabetes, Makyla said, "It seems to be taking forever, so I don't think it will happen until I'm older."

Makyla Sever, welcome to the Sisterhood of Diabetes. We embrace you and look forward to hearing about your successes in the future. ✂

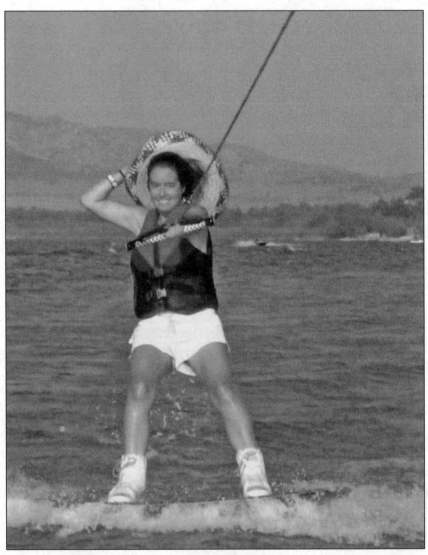

Jenny Vandevelde

JENNY VANDEVELDE
"C'mon! Let's Do It!"

Jenny was dressed in full soccer gear ready to practice with her team for an upcoming game. The co-ed team of eighteen year olds was highly competitive and Jenny was psyched to have made the team. She was fourteen years old.

On that day her mom drove her to the soccer field, stopping on the way for Jenny's routine required physical exam. When the doctor checked Jenny's blood sugar with a finger stick, she became concerned at the HI reading and strongly suggested they go to the hospital for further tests. "Can I go to soccer practice first?" Jenny cried. "It's off the same freeway exit."

At the hospital the doctors were amazed that all Jenny wanted to do was go play soccer when her blood glucose was over 800. In retrospect, the classic symptoms of thirst, blurry vision and weight loss were clearly present. During her four-day hospital stay, whenever the nurses were out of sight, Jenny played soccer in the hallways. The day after being released, she played in that momentous soccer game.

In the first few months following her diagnosis, her insulin schedule and soccer schedules collided head on. Jenny teetered between being too full at soccer and fighting low blood sugars. So she put her mind to researching a better way to make things work and she found it. She went on a Medtronic insulin pump two months after diagnosis and has been playing sports successfully ever since.

If It's Available … She'll Play It

Canyons of biking trails, soccer fields, jogging paths, lakes, basketball courts and endless sun surround Rancho Penasquitos in the northern island area of San Diego where Jenny grew up and calls home. If you want to go wakeboarding, it's a quick thirty-minute drive. Snowboarding is a two-hour drive that seems a hike for most people, but if you are Jenny Vandevelde, it's a carefree glide up the freeway while chatting with snowboarder friends and listening to lively music. Jenny is the wild, outdoorsy, perpetual-motion gal who everybody wants to hang out with. Her sports resume includes:

- *Gymnastics:* ages four through eleven, with a one-year hiatus at age seven due to a broken elbow from diving off a table.
- *Soccer:* Jenny discovered soccer while on a family trip to England when she was five years old. But it took her two years to convince her parents that she would not hit the ball with her head. She began playing on teams when she was eight. Soccer quickly became her favorite sport. She played highly competitive soccer throughout middle and high school years. Currently Jenny plays five to six times each week on five co-ed teams and one women's soccer team.
- *Ice Skating:* Skating coincided with soccer when Jenny was about five years old. It was a sport she enjoyed when she wasn't on the soccer field.
- *Basketball:* At eleven, a classmate suggested she might like basketball since she was such a good soccer player. Basketball soon replaced ice skating. She participated through middle and high school, playing on a co-ed team for two years during that period. Her position was point guard … and she had a great time taking on the boys.
- *Wakeboarding:* Jenny has lots of fun wakeboarding with friends in the San Diego area. This surface water sport that was started in 1980 combines water skiing, snowboarding and

surfing. Wakeboards are made of foam or honeycomb and resin and have a fiberglass coating. Metal screws attach fins and bindings. The rider is towed behind a motorboat or pulled by closed course cables at speeds of twenty to twenty-five mph. It is popular in lakes or on inter-coastal waterways.

- *Snowboarding:* At age seventeen, snowboarding became Jenny's sport *numero uno*. She believes that diabetes led her to it. One day, a flyer came in the mail advertising a one-day snowboarding camp for teens with diabetes. Sean Busby, a semi-pro Type 1 snowboarder was running the camp. Jenny called one of her fellow Type 1 buddies and off they went to Big Bear, California. Half way through the first day Jenny stood up on a board, glided down a hill and that was it—a love affair began. She went back the following year and became quite adept at maneuvering the board through hills of snow.

- *Running:* Running is a way for Jenny to keep in shape. After all, the best runner usually gets the ball in a soccer match, and whoever is in the best shape can do the most snowboarding runs. In 2008 Jenny was invited to run the Medtronic Twin Cities Marathon as a Medtronic Global Hero. The Global Heroes program, a cooperative effort between Twin Cities in Motion and the Medtronic Foundation recognizes runners from around the world who have a medical device to treat conditions such as diabetes. Every year twenty-five Global Heroes are selected from all over the world to run on the Global Hero team.

Cycling for Diabetes

Jenny has successfully completed two of the grueling JDRF (Juvenile Diabetes Research Foundation) Ride to Cure Diabetes cycling events in Death Valley. She rode with her dad both times. Shortly before the first ride in 2006, Jenny suffered a concussion. To complicate matters, her

In Jenny's Words

I was chosen for the Medtronic Global Heroes team based on my submission essay in May 2008, and immediately started a training program for the Minneapolis-St. Paul Marathon that is part of the Global Heroes program. I gradually increased my runs from 3-5 miles to 10-15 miles several times a week. I even ran pretty steep hills in 90-degree heat in the summer. After the runs I'd go to my soccer game.

The race was crazy. It began before sunrise with below freezing temperatures (not something I'm used to being from San Diego). I had inserted two insulin pump sites so that in case one went bad I would have a backup site to switch to. About three miles in, it started raining and I started feeling pretty sick. I tested my blood sugar and it was in the 500s. I took some insulin and kept going, hoping it would come down. I chugged as much water as possible at rest stops. At six miles I tested again to discover an over 600 (HI) reading on my meter. This pump site wasn't working for me. I switched to the other site. I kept running and the rain was running even faster, coming down so hard I could barely see. My contact lenses fogged up and my shoes were completely waterlogged. Every piece of clothing I wore was drenched. I was shivering. I struggled with the mind-over-matter aspect of how sick I felt and how cold I was when I spotted one of the other Global Heroes running by. She was an insulin-pumping diabetic just like me. She smiled and waved and I knew that I had to finish. I had to ignore the elements and the curveballs that diabetes was aiming at me. Suddenly that second wave of energy burst through and I crossed the finish line. I was immediately taken to the medical tent since I was purple. Apparently the 33 degree rain resulted in hypothermia. I could not even speak. But I had finished my first marathon and was so proud to have represented healthy diabetics that day and will never ever forget my incredible experience as a Global Hero.

blood glucose meter died from heat exhaustion in the 117-degree heat and she was at the mercy of other riders to check her blood sugar.

The first person she borrowed a meter from was a Canadian. In Canada they use a different number base of "mmol/dl" instead of the American set of "mg/dl." *Oops.* When the medics asked if she wanted a ride to the finish line, Jenny knew there was no way she would accept one. After all, she had raised $13,000 in donations from kids who set up lemonade stands for her after reading about her bike ride in the newspaper. She had donations from neighbors and others in her community. Her soccer team families gave donations and she had collected six hundred cell phones and recycled them to raise money; plus, companies such as Amylin and Pfizer gave money after she spoke to these organizations about diabetes and sports. She simply could not let herself and everyone down.

Jenny finished the ride. When she and her dad rode across the finish line, they couldn't have been happier or more proud. She was completely exhausted but beaming with joy. "The soles of my shoes had melted from a distinct orange and blue Nike to a shade of brown from the scorching asphalt we were on for those twelve hours."

The second Death Valley ride in October 2007 was also not without complications. Jenny remembers:

Less than twenty-four hours before the ride was supposed to start, my insulin pump died. I was thinking, "Oh no I'm in the middle of the desert about to bike for twelve hours and I have to go back to shots?!" I called Medtronic hoping they could help and they called me back thirty minutes later to say that a man named Javier would drive my new pump to Death Valley. I had the pump up and running just in time for dinner, and JDRF invited Javier to dinner in appreciation for all he did for me that day.

The next day the weather was no less brutal than during my first ride. Temperatures were more "mild" only topping out at *about 100 degrees, but we were faced with 40 mph winds with gusts up to 60 mph. It was so bad that I got knocked off my bike at least a dozen times from wind gusts. Sand was blowing everywhere and my eyes and throat were sucking it up. The worst part was the last uphill pull. I don't know how my dad and I made it, but we did. I was so excited to finish and to have ridden sixty-six miles that I immediately forgot all the elements that were working against me. Also I was grateful about the $11,000 in donations going to JDRF to get us closer to a cure.*

One of the big sources of donations came from a video I made with family and friends—a humorous tale about the difficulties of fundraising and training for the ride. The video was put on www. youtube.com and its popularity raised about $4,000 there.

Crutches

For someone as active in so many fast moving and competitive sports as Jenny is, tumbles sometimes occur, and she has had her share. The bumps and bruises, broken elbows and concussions of earlier years were nothing compared to the fall she took during a soccer game in 2010 when she fractured her talus bone (which connects the foot to the ankle to the leg). It happened on the date of her sixth anniversary of her diabetes diagnosis, and set Jenny reeling, putting her out of commission for over nine months. She was devastated physically and mentally from the severity of the pain and the slow healing prognosis of the fracture. Her best friend, her mom, stepped in to ease the burden, driving her to watch soccer games and always being available to talk about all the biggest and smallest problems in the world.

As Jenny recovered, she reflected on her life in sports and life with diabetes. She believes that being in the best shape you can is the best preparation for any activity. If not for diabetes, she would never would have cycled Death Valley two times or organized a team to walk the ADA Walk and raised over $30,000.

Diabetes makes me work harder to prove myself. Being a girl also makes me work hard to prove myself. And being a diabetic female I must prove myself against the non-diabetic males. Diabetes has made me tougher. A bruise or headache is not a big deal when you can give injections without batting an eyelash and you can avoid passing out from low blood sugars. I, for sure, have an "it's not going to stop me" attitude. Sometimes I have to carry extra supplies or figure out about disconnecting my pump, but there is no sport I cannot do because of diabetes.

Jenny volunteers as a counselor at Camp Wana Kura in Santee, California, and at Children With Diabetes conferences. She would like to work in the diabetes community in a position which involves outdoor and sports instruction when she graduates from San Diego State University where she is an A-student majoring in recreation systems management.

No doubt Jenny Vandevelde will be an asset to the diabetes community with her attitude of "Live life to its fullest. Love life and those you share your life with. Love everything you do."

The Sisterhood of Diabetes salutes you, Jenny Vandevelde! ✂

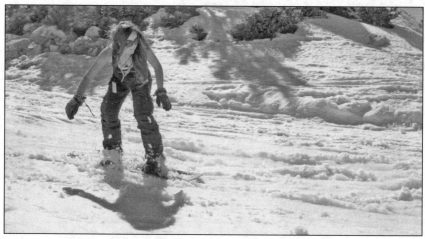

Jenny snowboards in California mountains

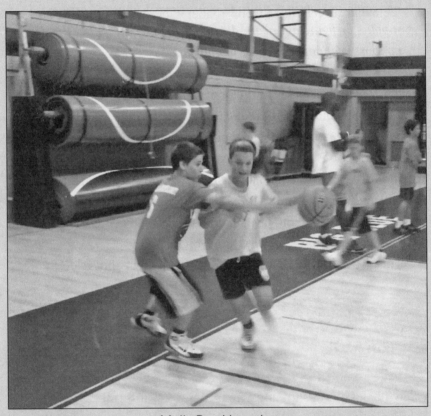

Molly Read in action

MOLLY READ

Shoots Hoops Around Diabetes

Molly was diagnosed at age ten, in 2007, but until that moment she had never heard the word "diabetes." Today she already thinks of her diabetes as a way of life.

Molly has a great network of support from family, friends at school, teammates and her diabetes team at the Naomi Berri Diabetes Center at New York Presbyterian Hospital. Diabetes makes her feel special, she says; she has to take on responsibilities that other kids her age don't know about, like being aware of where her blood sugar numbers are going, especially when she is playing basketball.

When she was diagnosed with diabetes, she thought to herself, "There is no way I'm *not* going to play basketball," the game she started playing in fourth grade and loves so much. During her years at Manasquan Elementary School, she even played for two different teams—her school team, Squan, where at five-foot-nine she was the tallest girl on the team, and in the Manasquan Mid-Monmouth basketball league which travels all over the large geographical area of Monmouth County. She also played a couple of seasons for an AAU team, the Jersey Shore Sharks.

During games, Molly distinguishes herself by setting up plays and sometimes going in for a basket wearing her signature red socks. She rarely misses a foul shot and dunks many to win games for her teams. While playing, Molly disconnects her Medtronic pump and CGM, but does lots of checking of blood sugars before, during and after events.

At her young age, Molly Read is already a champion and success story—both on the court and in school where she does well . . . math is her favorite subject. She is a role model for all the Sisterhood of Diabetes to look up to, admire, encourage and root for—on the basketball court and in her bright future. ✂

KAYLEY WOLF

Looks for Hurdles to Jump

Having been diagnosed with Type 1 diabetes at age four and learning how to give herself insulin shots might have something to do with how and why Kayley Wolf is so disciplined and committed. She has a clear memory of sitting in the pediatrician's office with her mom. When the doctor said, "Take her to Children's," Kayley was thrilled at the prospect of going to the "children's" playground. Little did she know he meant Cincinnati Children's Hospital where she would get her first insulin injection.

Kayley graduated *cum laude* from the best public high school in Ohio—Wyoming High School—as a National Honors Society member with a straight A average. The summer following graduation she interned in Washington D.C. on the JDRF [Juvenile Diabetes Research Foundation] Government Relations committee where, besides performing the routine tasks of any intern such as logging data entries and making copies, she worked with those making testimonies to Congress, including a spectrum of diabetes medical experts.

While on the committee, Kayley met Svati Nerula [another of the Sisters noted in this book], and together they created a brainstorming group which figured out projects, events and campaigns to appeal to the greatest numbers of Type 1 and Type 2 audiences.

As a student at Brandeis University in Boston, Kayley's studies in Public Health took her far and wide, including a research project in Arica, Chile.

An accomplished musician, Kayley has performed as a violinist in concerts in the U.S., Australia and the Czech Republic. She is a recipient of the Leonard Bernstein Scholarship. In addition, Kayley volunteers her musical talent at nursing homes and in hospitals.

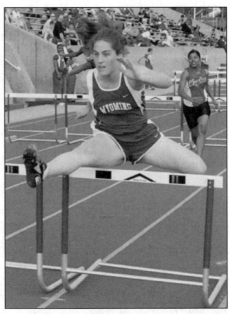

Kayley Wolf

Kayley Plays Sports!

The history of Kayley's life in sports runs all over the place. It's in her nature to be both athletic and competitive. As a youngster she was wild about soccer, gymnastics and basketball, and she loved the rough and tumble and challenge of playing sports with boys. (After attending the Chris Dudley Basketball Camp for kids with diabetes where she played basketball with "all guys" for five years as a camper, she went on to work as a counselor at the camp which she continues to do every year.) But sometimes the boys were threatened by her skills and powerful sense of competition. One time in fifth grade during a soccer match, Kayley scored against a boy who thought he was the greatest soccer player in town. He couldn't grasp the fact that a girl outscored him. As she was running across the field, he tripped her, causing a nasty ankle injury. Kayley got up and continued to bring her team home to victory. She still bears the "scars" from that injury.

Since girls were not allowed to officially play football, Kayley became a cheerleader. Cheerleading was quite athletic and fun for her since one of the qualities she loved most about sports was the camaraderie and sense of being a team player. But somewhere along the road in high school, this team player discovered a great passion—for sprinting and hurdling.

Kayley remembers speaking with the best runner in her school who had won numerous state championships; she held him up as a role model. As they spoke that day, he looked over at the track where a hurdler was going through the rigors of training. He shook his head and said, "Those hurdlers are crazy. I could never do that." This was all Kayley had to hear. Next day she was on the field full out in her first hurdling practice!

Diabetes, Life and Sports

Like all the other Sisters in this book, Kayley deals with the double challenge of competing in sports and pushing through her diabetes. When her blood glucose numbers are stable, it's clear sailing and excellence all the way to first place. Unfortunately, much of the diabetes part is out of her control.

Kayley found that college track events presented so many variables that it was sometimes difficult to stabilize blood sugars. First, there is the "nervous factor" before races. Add to that, the mix of sprinting and distance running, as well as trying to take in the right nutrition leading up to events. But, through luck and an ample amount of research, Kayley was able to run for her university track team and to train with 2008 Olympic silver-medal winner David Payne (from the University of Cincinnati) in the 110 meter hurdles,. This inspiring athlete was interested and helpful in coaching Kayley to improve her natural talents as a sprinter and hurdler.

A Family Affair

Kayley grew up in a strong family environment and treasures her close ties with her mom, dad and brother. Her mother, a former ballet dancer and model and current aerobics instructor, is a very active JDRF volunteer who has chaired the Cincinnati JDRF Gala many times and helped raise millions of dollars for diabetes research. Kayley's dad is an airline

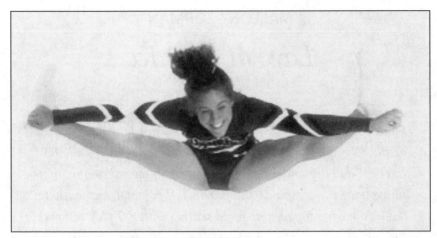

Kayley flies

captain and graduate of the United States Air Force Academy. He too has worked tirelessly JDRF projects. Her older brother, who happens to also be one of her very best friends, is an officer in the Coast Guard with plans to go to medical school when he leaves the service. Kayley told me, "I have always looked at my family as pretty much perfect human beings." She hesitates with a smile, "Even though they definitely know how to embarrass me."

Diabetes is with Kayley Wolf day in and day out. She has spoken with many friends who also have diabetes and they all agree diabetes has a great influence on how they shape their lives. She told me,

I think that is part of the reason diabetics are drawn to each other. It is a special disease unlike any other. Most of the work is in the hands of the patients. Being an athlete with diabetes is twice as hard as being an athlete without diabetes, but the reward is twice as great.

Thanks, Kayley Wolf, for being such an outstanding Sister! 🦋

MALLORY ZORMAN

Love at First Ice

From September to March every year I train four days a week at the Olympic Oval in Calgary in both long track and short track . . . and dryland program. I compete in several competitions throughout the season at the provincial, regional and national level. Following my regular speed skating season, I play competitive soccer, participate in speed skating dryland activities and train for and compete in cross country running. I also like to roller blade and bike on the trails around my home. I spend one week every summer at an intense speed-skating training camp.

Mallory Zorma has her eyes set on winning a medal in the Olympics one day! She has already won acclaim in her native Canada—in 2007 Mallory won Bronze in the 2007 Nationals; in 2009 she was part of the relay team that won the silver medal in the Canadian Speed Skating Nationals.

Mallory was awarded the Desa Youth Athletic Achievement Award at an international Diabetes, Exercise and Sports Association conference in 2006 in Toronto. To qualify for this honor, she had to submit an essay, excerpted below. I think you will enjoy reading it.

Managing diabetes and sports can be a tough thing. Speed skating is a sport where it's very tough to manage blood sugar levels because it includes distances that are both sprints and endurance. I've found that I get my best results when my blood sugar is in good control. When I train with high blood sugar, I feel tired and have less energy. I have also experienced being low while racing. I work really hard at testing a lot during training and competitions and balancing my food and insulin.

On top of being very busy with skating, I work really hard at school and maintain a 96-percent average. I really like biology, math and P.E. School remains a strong aspect of my life and I want to continue to get good grades and go on to university.

Mallory Zorman is obviously out there in the front line with those women who make a positive difference in the world. The accomplishments are already adding up for this young Sister ... and no doubt there will be many more in her future.   ❧

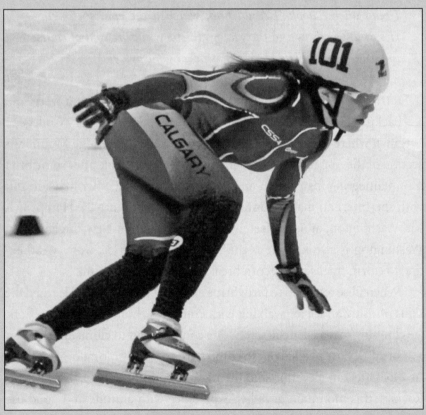

Mallory Zorman

ELISE ZEVITZ

Climbing to the Top on Insulin Power

I read all the books I could find, watched the epic documenta-
ries and was drawn to the geology, history, culture and of course,
mountaineering. The interest has never gone away.

Starting in 2008, Elise began rock climbing three times a week and backpacking with the climbing club at William and Mary College in Virginia, where she was a student. She hiked the Blue Ridge Mountains section of the Appalachian Trail and during spring break, after some brief mountaineering instruction and gear rental, she made her first summit with the International Mountain Climbing School in New Hampshire. Mt. Washington, at 6,288 feet, is the highest peak in New England. Mt. Washington is also known as the "home of the world's worst weather," due to storm tracks and record breaking winds of 231 mph.

When Elise returned to terra firma after that climb, she had learned the skills of using an ice ax, walking with crampons, building snow anchors, ice climbing and avalanche safety. She couldn't wait to climb again.

In 2009, Elise headed out to climb to the roof of Colorado, Mt. Elbert. At 14,433 feet in elevation and the highest point in the North American Rockies, this mountain gave her experience with altitude and good use of the skills she had learned in New Hampshire. Besides the adventure

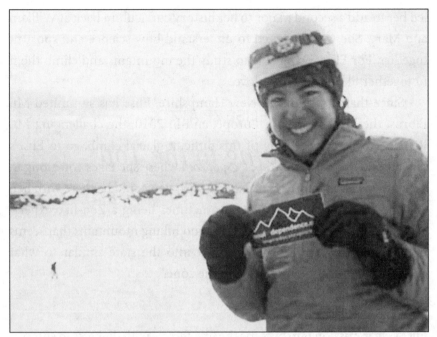

Elise Zevitz, at the summit

and thrill of mountaineering, Elise quickly learned by trial and error the basic skills of climbing mountains with diabetes. She learned not to trust her normal feelings of high or low blood sugars. In the mountains, your blood glucose might be low when you think you're high or it could simply be altitude or fatigue; the symptoms are all similar when you're climbing high. It's all about checking blood sugars often, and being willing to adapt to life in high altitudes and the sometimes quirky dictates of Mother Nature. It means keeping your blood glucose meter insulated and close to your body so it doesn't catch a cold. Mountain climbing is a very strenuous, very aerobic sport and requires frequent carbohydrate fueling.

The more Elise got to know and love mountaineering, she realized it was not only the experience of being outdoors and the adventure and beauty of nature that fascinated her. It was also a strong sense of inquisitiveness about the process and timescale of how mountains form and the scientific forces at work that she wanted to know more about. This led her to add a second major to her history curriculum back at William and Mary. She was intrigued to understand how science and sport fit together. For Elise, being able to study the mountains and climb them fit together like a hand in a glove.

Since that first climb in New Hampshire, Elise has summited Mt. Elbrus, the highest peak in Europe, and in 2010, the challenging Mt. Rainer. To share something of this difficult glacial climb, go to Elise's blog, *www.climbingoninsulin.blogspot.com* where she takes you along in vivid words and pictures, making you wish you could be there with her. She describes mountaineering as sometimes being a Zen-like experience. There is a tranquility in walking and hiking mountains that seems nomadic and rhythmic when you get into the state similar to what runners call the "runner's high" or "the zone."

Onward and Upward

Elise's clear mission is to become the first female with diabetes to summit the seven tallest peaks in the world, known as the Seven Summits. This would also make her the first woman with diabetes to reach the top of the world, Mt. Everest.

Diabetes management is in a state of change now, some may say it is a revolutionary time and it is this generation of inspiration who are paving the way for the future of possibilities. As Elise Zevitz says so eloquently in her blog:

> *I believe women with diabetes can do anything and I want to inspire my generation to take an active and dynamic role in beating diabetes. In this way, I hope to inspire people with or without diabetes to reach for the summit of their own Everest.*

Kudos to you Elise, and your powerful family of diabetes sisters who are raising the bar for the now and next generation of those who live with diabetes. This is your time!   🦋

Special thanks to the shining stars in this book who continue to enlighten, motivate and inspire all those who live with diabetes.

Acknowledgements

Inspiration is a gift. I feel blessed by the gift of having been inspired by the sisters who told me their stories. They are role models for all of us. Everyone whose story lives within these pages has brought energy, excitement and awareness of the importance of a positive attitude and the possibilities of dreams coming true.

Without encouragement and technical assistance from my husband and partner in life, Danny Ambrosini, the book might not have been completed. It was his seamless support that taught me confidence and endurance.

From the get-go, my best and brilliant friend from high school days in Schenectady, New York, Maureen Brunner, assigned herself as editor a la minute. She ferociously red penciled her way through my sometimes too wordy sentences.

Continuous support from Joanie Middleton-Mahon, Elaine O'Brien, Nancy Pongrac, Bill King, Ruth Roberts, John Walsh, Max Szadek, Noreen Davidson, Charles Renfroe, Victor Van Beuren, Riva Greenberg, Chris Zullo, Jill and Jude Sheehan bolstered my focus and energy throughout the book's journey. Sheri Colberg-Ochs is the friend and seasoned author who helped steer me through the labyrinth of publishing.

Thank you Hohm-Kalindi Press for your belief and understanding in *The Sisterhood of Diabetes.* I wish to acknowledge my wise woman editor, Regina Sara Ryan, the stranger who became a friend and sister during the process.

I thank every person in the diabetes community who has sparked my passion about the importance of staying active, motivated to move and forging a kinship with diabetes.

And thank you Thomas Dove Ambrosini Sheehan, age seven, for inspiring the powerful by-line, "Facing Challenges & Living Dreams."

Suggested Reading

Biermann, June and Barbara Toohey, *The Diabetic's Sports & Exercise Book*. Philadelphia and New York: J.B. Lippincott Company, 1977.

Colberg, Sheri PhD, *Diabetic Athlete's Handbook*. Illinois: Human Kinetics. 2008

_____, *The 7 Step Diabetes Fitness Plan: Living Well and Being Fit with Diabetes, No Matter Your Weight* (Marlowe Diabetes Library); Boston: Da Capo Press, 2005.

_____, *The Diabetic Athlete*. Illinois: Human Kinetics, 2001.

Cooper, Thea and Arthur Ainsberg, *Breakthrough: Elizabeth Hughes, the Discovery of Insulin, and the Making of a Medical Miracle*. New York: St. Martin's Press, 2010.

Dudley, Chris, *Chris Dreams BIG*. CCD Productions, 2009.

Edelman, Steven V. MS, *Taking Control of Your Diabetes*. New York: Professional Communications, Inc.3rd Edition, 2007.

Greenberg, Riva, *Diabetes Do's & How-To's: Small yet powerful steps to take charge, eat right, get fit and stay positive*. New York: Professional Communications, Inc. 2013

Jovanovic, Lois MD, *Managing Your Gestational Diabetes: A Guide for You and Your Baby's Good Health*. Hoboken, N.J.: John Wiley & Sons, 1994.

Karz, Zippora, *The Sugarless Plum: A Memoir*. Ontario, Canada: Harlequin, 2011.

Ruderman, Neil ed., *Handbook of Exercise in Diabetes*. Alexandria, Virginia: American Diabetes Association, 2002.

Scheiner, Gary, MS, CDE, *Think Like a Pancreas: A Practical Guide to Managing Diabetes with Insulin* (Completely Revised and Updated). Boston: Da Capo Lifelong Books, 2012.

Schuller, Catherine, *The Ultimate Plus-Size Modeling Guide.* Emerging Visions Enterprises. 1997

Southerland, Phil, *Not Dead Yet: My Race Against Disease: From Diagnosis to Dominance.* New York: Thomas Dunne Books, 2011.

Thurm, Ulrike, *CGM–und Insulinpumpenfibel.* Germany: Kirchheim + Co. GmbH; 2. Auflage, 2013. Language: German

Thurm, Ulrike, *Diabetes–und Sportfibel: Mit Diabetes weiter laufen.* Germany: *Kirchheim + Co. GmbH* 01.2008. Language: German

Vieira, Ginger, *Your Diabetes Science Experiment: Live your live with diabetes, instead of letting diabetes live your life.* CreateSpace Independent Publishing Platform, 2012.

Walsh, John P.A., CDE and Roberts, Ruth M.A., *Pumping Insulin: Everything You Need to Succeed on an Insulin Pump.* San Diego, Calif.: Torrey Pines Press, 5th edition 2012.

_____, *Using Insulin: Everything You Need for Success with Insulin.* San Diego, Calif.: Torrey Pines Press, 2003.

Index

About the Author

JUDITH JONES-AMBROSINI has lived under the influence of Type 1 diabetes since 1962. Diabetes has guided her down many winding roads and pathways, one of which has led to involvement and advocacy for empowering those with diabetes through sports and exercise. She herself is a distance walker. Her first marathon was in Denmark in 2005. She walks the 32-mile rim of Manhattan Island every spring, and is a dedicated proponent and practitioner of daily exercise including dance, strength training, cycling, gardening, flexibility/balance as well as being a teacher and practitioner of t'ai chi. Judith has been writing about food, healthy lifestyle and diabetes for newspapers, magazines and websites since 1992. She lives with her husband and family in Greenwich Village, NY and spends getaway time in a small quiet town on the Jersey Shore. *The Sisterhood of Diabetes* is her first book.

Contact information: *diabetesmotivation@gmail.com*
website: *www.thesisterhoodofdiabetes.com*

About Kalindi Press

KALINDI PRESS, an affiliate of **HOHM PRESS**, proudly offers books in natural health and nutrition, as well as the acclaimed *Family Health* and *World Health Series* for children and parents, covering such themes as nutrition, dental health, reading, and environmental education.

Contact: *hppublisher@cableone.net*
Visit our website at: *www.kalindipress.com*